"My first experience of re_ _ _ _ _ _ _ _ _ _ was profound, and I have been hooked ever since. I have been involved in body work for many years and have had hundreds of body work sessions internationally. What makes Wayne's sessions so profound is the depth he takes me to and the magic that gets evoked for weeks after my sessions. I literally feel all old baggage fall off, injuries healing fast, and my energy shiny, new, and ready to take on the world from a place of heart and soul. I now make receiving Wayne's healing work part of my lifestyle and a must for my family and the clients I mentor. I urge you to experience, learn, and dive into Wayne's magic and I assure you that you'll be gifting yourself a spa-healing for your body, mind, and soul."

—Satyen Raja, founder of Warrior Sage Trainings

"… The mature lomilomi practitioner, no matter the franchise, always lives within the current of authority to heal. The core relationship between the soul and the practitioner is the maturing process. When that happens; the healing that follows is immortal. The place we hold for lomilomi is far reaching, so many practitioners have far moved past the certificates on their wall and into their own expression. In that expression is the non-franchised, authentic relationship between soul and person, carrying the healing that is known as lomilomi. And Wayne and Patti's effort in this book speaks to all lineages in a single voice."

—Harry Uhane Jim, Kahuna, healer, teacher, and author of *Wise Secrets of Aloha*

"Many are the techniques for revitalizing and relaxing the body temple, but there is only one that delivers the results of Wayne's Lomilomi techniques. Wayne's unique combination of Lomilomi and ancient breath work promotes the integration of healthy new choices while releasing old ones. In short it is a transforming gift to yourself!"

—Rev. Dr. Michael Bernard Beckwith,
founder and senior minister of Agape International
Spiritual Centre, and author of *Life Visioning*

HAWAIIAN
SHAMANISTIC
HEALING

About the Authors

Wayne Kealohi Powell, DD, a Doctor of Divinity, weaves his experiences and qualifications as a motivational speaker, author, reverend, Lomilomi and Touch for Health instructor, Alakai (minister) of the Order of Huna International, singer/songwriter, and recording artist/producer into his life's offering as a Holistic Health educator. He is the founder and senior Instructor of Shamanic Bodywork, an educational vehicle focusing on the highest wisdom of the human soul's ability to heal cherished wounds and restore its "original innocence," reclaiming its birthright to be healthy and abundant in all things.

His training in various healing modalities with Serge Kahili King, Abraham Kawai'i, Sherman Dudoit, Harry Uhane Jim, John deRuiter, Wayne Topping, and Glenda Green have become the formula for the global success of his work and has earned him the title "Midwife of the soul." Invitations to spread his healing wings have seen him travel and teach for more than two decades throughout the United States and Canada, Costa Rica, Fiji, Australia, Europe, and the United Kingdom.

Wayne believes in the strength of the human spirit (as an aspect of God) to redeem its own perfection through ho'oponopono—radical forgiveness and the power of blessing. His practice is holistic as he works to resolve the misalignments within the trinity of body, mind, and spirit as a cluster of souls. Wayne has assisted many to transform their suffering and pain into a peaceful, renewed relationship to life, through authenticating accountability of the natural harmony within their soul cluster.

Patricia Lynn Miller is a vehicle for spiritual energy, embodying the aloha spirit with great artistic flare. Her academic education was in Fine Arts, studying painting, life drawing, sculpture, printmaking, and illustration at Georgian College in Ontario, Canada. Her further education lead her to undertake Aboriginal Studies (Native Spirituality), which included chanting, pipe carrying (how to use tobacco as a sacred healing medicine), sweat lodge teachings, and ceremonial healing work. She has practiced shamanic healing, reiki, and Wiccan spirituality. She is a medicine woman specializing in aromatherapy and therapeutic essential oils. It is Hawaiian healing that has been her true main focus. She studied Temple Style lomi and kahuna science with Wayne Powell, Heartworks lomi with Sherman Dudoit, Aunty Margaret style lomi with Kim and Jim Hartley, Hawaiian healing with Harry Uhane Jim, ho'oponopono with Lawrence Kamani Aki and Harry Uhane Jim, Hawaiian protocol, history, and crafts with Anakala Pilipo Solatorio, Hawaiian hula and music with Dhyana Ahiwai Bartkow, and Lono's halau on Molokai. Patti is a born nurturer. She is an artist in the kitchen and loves to create food for people. She is a seasoned recording artist with the voice of an angel who is also quite passionate about writing and illustrating children's books.

Visit her website at www.shamanicbodywork.com.

HAWAIIAN SHAMANISTIC HEALING

Medicine Ways to
Cultivate the Aloha Spirit

WAYNE KEALOHI POWELL
PATRICIA LYNN MILLER

Llewellyn Worldwide
Woodbury, Minnesota

FIRST EDITION
First Printing, 2018

Book design by Bob Gaul
Cover design by Kevin R. Brown
Figure drawings on pages 261–262 by Mary Ann Zapalac and
Llewellyn art department

Llewellyn Publications is a registered trademark of Llewellyn Worldwide Ltd.

Library of Congress Cataloging-in-Publication Data (Pending)
ISBN: 978-0-7387-5049-1

Llewellyn Publications
A Division of Llewellyn Worldwide Ltd.
2143 Wooddale Drive
Woodbury, MN 55125-2989
www.llewellyn.com

Printed in the United States of America

CONTENTS

DEDICATION

To all those who carry knowledge of the sacred, the wise ones who share it with humility and compassion, and to everyone who has assisted another to feel comfort and kindness when they needed it most, we honor you and bless you.

To our family and extended family—especially Wayne's children: Jarod, Colon, Ethan, and their mother: Jana; Patti's daughter Ariana, and Wayne's granddaughter Alessia—may you all receive the utmost benefit from this work of love. And to all our unknown ancestors and descendants: may all your prayers be answered.

Big mahalo to all our teachers who inspired and awakened the ancient rhythms of Aloha Spirit within us: this book is the fruit of our steadfast devotion to you, in the honoring of ourselves, acknowledging what is sacred within all of us and blessing everyone who comes to us. Mahalo 'Aumakua for guiding our personal mission of healing through Aloha—the Breath of God, as spiritual intimacy.

INTRODUCTION

You are needed! In choosing to take up this book, you embark on an assignment to bring forth memories of an ancient wisdom. Deep within you is a unique medicine that only you carry, an inner knowing of your purpose here on Earth. It is time for all of you to answer the call to share your medicine, and reinstate the value of human existence at the forefront of creation in these changing times. You've been in training for lifetimes and did not come unprepared. All you need to know is inside you, and now your task is to remember. This is the great awakening and everyone is involved. This is our journey together, for we are our own salvation. You are an important member of the family; you came to Earth at this time as an advocate of healing to embrace the paradox and unify polarities, release the fear of being alone, and remember and reclaim your universal birthright—original innocence.

The calling to become a shaman or miracle worker emerges from deep within your soul, and yet this calling is also from nature for your soul to remember its purpose here. It may feel like a loud and clear message, or it may just be a quiet curiosity that slowly grows over time. But know that either way, this is your higher self guiding you to a greater understanding of life and your place in existence. Each person and every aspect of life is irreplaceable. What you bring to the Earth no one else will. The path of each shaman is unique. It's a journey of self-discovery that arises out of inner promptings that often lead you into very dark places, which are yearning to receive more light through you. We all are given the capacity to forgive, transforming fearful and hurtful feelings into connections of unity with all life. We address and release them within ourselves first and then assist others to do likewise.

This book was written to inspire and open your heart by offering a long, fresh breath of pure *aloha* (unconditional love and grace) to facilitate your healing journey. It's not intended as a completed treatise on Hawaiian shamanism, bodywork, traditions, or cultural practices. Rather it is a collection of conscious spiritual ideas, practices, and philosophy, coupled with effective bodywork techniques. If you try the many exercises and healing techniques contained in the pages here, you will find that you learn a whole new way of relating to your body. By learning how to communicate with the wisdom of your body, you may tap into your own intuition and unlock your unlimited power and healing energy. You can also develop a relationship with the spirit world and become acquainted with your own spirit guides or guardian angels. You can release your inner shaman with trust, and create meaningful healing experiences for yourself and others.

What is being shared here on these pages has been created for the purpose of spreading aloha light to as many souls as possible for the healing of our global *'ohana* (family). Understanding how thoughts and vibrations influence the movement of our energy is advantageous to opening portals for healing and reshaping your reality. The teachings contained herein are seeds of ancient, cosmic knowledge here to provide you with the tools required to form shamanic relationships, navigating them in a conscious way that will benefit all humanity.

A'ohe pau ka 'ike i ka halau ho'okahi:
All knowledge is not taught in the same school

This is a presentation of Hawaiian bodywork techniques and medicine ways and the shamanic approach to life and healing. There are several shamanic rituals and ceremonial processes included for your enjoyment that were developed over a period of more than twenty-five years of studying, teaching classes, and seeing clients for private sessions. Wayne (Kealohi) created a five-hour healing session that combines the following processes: footbath, blessing with oils, sacred ceremonies for honoring the soul, ho'oponopono, truth dialog, spinal alignment, digestive system rebalancing, lomi ha breath medicine, and lomilomi massage. The healing processes in this book will introduce you to these aspects of our work so that you can begin to use them as a way to heal yourself and others.

We have been truly blessed over the years to have known, loved, and promoted masters of Hawaiian mysticism, shamanism, and healing traditions. Each of our teachers sustains a unique message of aloha spirit, rich in wisdom and practical application. In sharing the philosophy, knowledge, and healing techniques of these masters, our hope is that you, too, may drink the nectar of their wisdom among these pages and have it bear fruit in the garden of your own life. It truly is miraculous to witness the spreading of *ke aloha o ke Akua* (the Grace of God) through all the past and all the future generations to come. In the following pages, we will refer to these teachers in Hawaiian terms:

- *Kahu*: honored attendant, guardian, nurse, keeper of bones, clan caretaker, master, reverend, warden

- *Kumu*: instructor, teacher of cultural traditions and medicine ways: hula, lomilomi, weaving, ho'oponopono

- *Kupua*: one possessing *mana*, spiritual power, and influence (in modern terms—a shaman)

- *Kahuna*: priest, minister, master of a specific body and frequency of knowledge

+ *Uncle* or *Aunty*: the term of endearment for a
  respected, wise, and knowledgeable elder in one's
  life and community

The methods inspired by these teachers can provide profound opening, offer permanent change, and evoke higher qualities of living into action.

We share these methods to inspire and perhaps assist you to learn, generate, and allow profound miracles to take place for you and others around you in need of effective healing at this time. Miraculous things are happening every moment of our lives; it's all about becoming aware enough to recognize them and bless them when they occur.

And so it is with the utmost respect for the Hawaiian culture, their heritage and healing traditions, their land, and their way of life that we present *Hawaiian Shamanistic Healing* as living aloha medicine to facilitate your journey as a radiant "human beaming," and for the healing of your loved ones and your community. In honoring the tradition of Ho'oponopono, we must say: *E—kala mai ia'u!*

If we have offended anyone, their ancestors, or their descendants in any way by presenting here what has been our healing journey, we are truly sorry. Please forgive us.

May the warm wind of aloha blow through your soul and lift you above all the painful challenges of life, offering you divine purpose and a peace beyond understanding.

Me ke aloha pume hana ... With warm regards,
—Rev. Wayne Kealohi Powell, DD,
   and Patricia Lynn Kale'aokalani Miller

1

A Healer's Journey

Noho ka ikaika i ke aloha o ke Akua:
Our strength resides in the Grace of Divinity

The Calling

Deeper spiritual growth calls to many of us from within a passionate quest. Our calling is a personal journey, leading us to study many different cultures and approaches to effective healing. In our search for meaning and connection, we often look to cultures that have preserved their traditions to learn from the wisdom of those who have dedicated their lives to learning how to use the gifts of nature in a way that connects to a higher power. The Hawaiian culture offers many forms of healing that can be applied in a sacred way. One of the forms of healing Hawaii offers to the world is called *lomilomi*. The word *lomi* means massage as a noun, and lomilomi refers to the action of massaging as a verb. At first glance, lomilomi seems to be just a massage, but as we look deeper we see that it is much more—a process of soul evolution, a transformation that takes place on many levels and dimensions. For this reason, many people are called to it as a form of holistic medicine.

If you are feeling at all called to explore the world of the shaman or kahuna, it is because perhaps your soul is wanting to engage and grow into a higher purpose. When you respond or surrender to your soul's calling to evolve through a path of spiritual service, you will be forever changed in ways you cannot imagine. For some, it feels like a mystical hurricane scooping them up, threshing (like wheat), turning them inside out. It may feel like your whole world is falling apart, but if you surrender to the process, become humble and vulnerable, everything unforgiven (all unhealed issues) begin to surface for healing. With patience and compassion leading the way, everything changes for the better in time because in order to grow and evolve, we must face our fears. You will be presented with challenges but you will never be given more than you can handle. In facing your fears and overcoming those challenges, you will open up to experience greater love and greater power than you have ever felt before.

Be warned: your life may come completely unglued so that *ke Akua* (God or Spirit) can reassemble it in a manner that will make you more accessible and available to assist others to find their way as you have. This is love's promise—you will heal as you assist others to heal. This is spiritual law and not an adventure for the faint-hearted. It is a journey without a destination.

You do not have to wait until you are perfect to begin healing others. You can begin right now, from wherever you are in your development, to share your light, and light the way for others. Many "way showers" are being called right now to assist in the emotional maturing of humankind, and all your gifts are needed at this time.

Preparing for the Journey

Like many things in life, we realize there is no absolute way to prepare for the intense journey of self-healing and the healing of others. Healing is a journey without end, a process of maturing each individual soul as well as the collective human soul, balancing what's gone before with what's to come, in the here and now. This process continues long after the body is laid to rest. Healing is done through a trance state, which promotes and allows divine light to enter wherever needed. The best form of preparation is a daily spiritual practice that balances your body, mind, and spirit, and anchors you in a resilient Peace. When you take time each day to call more light to share space with you, there will be change. Light affects everything, and when a profound transformation that creates an unexpected yet desired result takes place, we call it a miracle. Where love as light has reclaimed its natural place, harmony and peace will always follow.

Challenges, Initiations, and Core Beliefs

Becoming a healer is a path of spiritual intimacy. This intimacy takes place first and foremost between you and the divine. Over time, the devoted healer learns to trust the unknowable good that breathes life into everything in existence. Before the arrival of mature artistry, there are many tests—of character, strength, and courage—that require you to be an attentive, loving light within all circumstance. In this way, every challenge becomes an initiation into a greater love. And it is by passing through these internal and external challenges that you become rooted in the landscape of your authentic self—as divine love—residing within an ever-increasing current of synchronicity and serendipity in the human experience.

Managing Beliefs Promotes Trust

Your personal beliefs are your blind spots to higher consciousness. When you hold a belief, it becomes a limited container for a personal experience. Radical ideas outside of your belief structure will cause you to feel unsafe—invalidated. No one feels safe when their beliefs are being challenged, and some feel very threatened and can become quite violent when this happens. It is for this reason people who believe in the same things hang out together—this way, their beliefs are not challenged. As a miracle worker, you will learn how to adjust your beliefs in order to get the results you are seeking. To be too attached to your beliefs would limit your effectiveness as a conduit for infinite Spirit. A kahuna in ancient times was trained to allow their beliefs to be adapted in each moment so that abundant mana could flow from Spirit unimpeded. It's a good idea to first examine your own core beliefs when doing your daily spiritual practice. You should also enquire about the core beliefs of those who come to you for help. Doing this will allow you to better facilitate an effective movement of healing energy. Basic psychology has shown us that all healing begins with a change in our thinking and our beliefs. This is also a very effective holistic medicine practice, because our experiences are filtered through and goverend by our personal beliefs.

Your world is what you think it is. What you believe in will become the pathway through which your healing will be expressed. You may want to begin speaking to yourself in a way that is unfamiliar to you, to unlock your psyche and reach a higher truth that brings the shift you want to experience. When you come across a belief pattern that is not serving you, we suggest you change it into a more effective one by following the gravity of love without conditions. You must examine your core beliefs because no healing can take place without the cooperation of the subconscious. When you repeat a new pattern, your subconscious will accept it as reality. You may attract certain circumstances in life that may lead you to a particular thought complex or core belief holding pain or negative emotions in place. Once you find it, unwind it and let it go. Then you will attract different circumstances into your life.

Core beliefs can range from "the world is a dangerous place" to "the world is a loving place" and "I will never amount to anything" to "I will achieve my dreams—I embrace success as my birthright." Each one of these beliefs will cause a very different behavior from the beholder and will in turn attract and animate a very different experience of life. Our limiting beliefs become our challenges. They stand as the structured posts that hold up the fence of our fears. When our beliefs are challenged, our need for control kicks in, and we look for ways to validate or defend our coveted beliefs and limiting understandings. If, however, we allow ourselves to drop our barriers, we can discover the hidden and underlying fear behind all those defenses. Once the root fear is brought to light, everything begins to change.

EXERCISE: Examine Your Limiting Beliefs

Ask yourself right now: which of your core beliefs are limiting you? Listen very carefully. Take a piece of paper and down one side write all the limiting beliefs that come to you on a regular basis. Be sure to write down at least one belief for each category: Career, Love, Money, Myself, World. Write down what you hear as well as the date you heard it. You may be surprised what comes up. On the other side of the page, write a more positive belief to read over and over whenever you think of it. Do this once a week for six weeks, and write down your experience as you feel a shift in your perceptions. Can you see how your personal beliefs change throughout your life as you mature spiritually? Many of the things that were so important to you ten years ago are not important now. Can you see how your beliefs that you are holding right now may actually be limiting your perception of yourself and others? Beliefs naturally create judgments and where judgment is, love cannot flow.

As you read this book, become aware of your thought processes. Focus your awareness on examining where you have been leaking your precious energy or holding back your creativity. Notice how every thought you have influences your direct experience of life. In time, you may discover which of your personal beliefs are limiting your capacity for navigating and maintaining a full conscious connection with your highest wealth, as precious love in a physical body. With practice, you will live in the knowing that your love for life will carry you through anything. You will be able to adjust your thinking in any given situation life brings, like becoming a good surfer: you learn to ride the more intensely challenging waves, take greater and greater risks, expand into ecstatic communion with the forces of nature, in love with the radical; perpetual motion through devotion!

Accepting Your Destiny

In ancient Hawaii, sometimes before a child was born, the parents or grandparents would be given visions or signs when a master was preparing to enter this plane of existence. Other times, through careful observation of the child at a very young age, they would know when the soul was ready to develop its gifts. They would present the youth to different aunties, uncles, and *kupuna* (respected elders), for training in various fields of expertise, activating their intuitive skills. Think about your own life for a moment. If someone had observed you as a child, what gifts would they have seen? What talents would they have helped you develop? These are keys to your destiny and clues to discovering your purpose here on Earth. It is time to honor yourself, fully develop those gifts, and bring them out into the world. Take a look at the talents you have that are just waiting to be shared. Look inside your heart and ask yourself what you are longing to do in this life. Your destiny will become clear and you will be guided as you begin to let go of the limitations you have placed upon yourself.

Trust the Process

Life on Earth is a precious gift to behold. A magnificent, flowering matrix of pure light from the heart of creation resides within each of us, and we all get to play in this beautiful garden together. Of course, life does not always look or feel so beautiful. The journey of a shaman or healer is a most exquisite one in which the activity of trust becomes our most valuable attribute to cultivate in order to survive the many challenges that will forge our faith, give us strength, and teach us how to thrive in love along the way. Of course you can never really fail, because you will always learn something about yourself through every choice you make, when you are truly being observant.

There is always value in feeling, remembering, knowing, and learning to *allow* what's occurring, in every moment of our lives. Resistance to what is, brings pain and suffering. Trusting the universal life source to look out for you, in all circumstances, brings peace. When we were in the womb, everything was provided for us; all our needs were met. It is important to remember that this support continues every day of our lives. In any moment, we can return to a safe place in our heart. We can find refuge from the chaos of the world through meditation, experiencing personal communion with the divine source of all life as our immortal soul. The mystic Osho said, "If you are having trouble finding your heart, just go to a cliff and jump! It will start beating so fast, it will be easy to find!"

Now let's look at what it takes to become a miracle worker and how to create a space for healing miracles in your life and the lives of others. By "miracle," we are referring to a substantial shift in perception (mind) from fear to love that brings one's body back into alignment with one's divinity (spirit). This shift takes place internally, creating dramatic results in the external world. Things come into alignment and you begin to become aware of the next step on the path of your true purpose. When you fully commit to the healer's journey, you may come to recognize and expect miracles every moment of your life. Yet, the miraculous is simply the extraordinary process of life revealed through a pure, innocent perception of what was already there.

▽△▽△▽△▽△▽△▽△▽△▽△▽△▽

EXERCISE: Open to Miracle-Mindedness

To Prepare: You can open to miracles now by learning to practice innocent perception. This exercise is to be done each morning upon rising and each evening when getting ready for sleep. It is a short meditation that can be done easily in any quiet location.

To begin: Innocent perception is achieved through courage and strength, because you must find a way to see beyond illusions, to look beneath the surface, and trust your higher self to guide you to a new way of viewing things. To practice innocent perception, begin the day by facing the sun and raising your hands, palms open. Ask to recognize the miracles of that day. When the day is done and you lay your head on the pillow at night, recall every miracle that you witnessed that day as you entered each situation. We suggest that you open your heart to the fact that you are in partnership with an infinite source of supply living through you that exists in and around all things. This is good—very good, indeed!

Shamanism and Kahuna Science

Due to today's environmental changes and the ever-accelerating shifts in human consciousness, more and more people from all walks of life are discovering access to previously hidden realms. In order for us to thrive or even survive, all of us are looking for a way of viewing the world that offers us a cooperative influence to circumstances and relationships, just like the shamans of old.

> *Ahuwale ka nane huna: That which*
> *was a secret is no longer hidden*
> —Mary Kawena Pukui

What Is a Shaman?

A shaman is someone who has a profound connection with nature and the ability to interact with the natural elements in such ways as to create a shift in perception of reality. Each shaman has a specific body of knowledge that they learn to master and use to elicit change, such as the use of plant medicine, psychic abilities, working in the dream state or other dimensions, or the art of sacred ceremony. A shaman has the intuitive ability to see the unseen and hear the unspoken. This can include communicating with the spirits of people who have passed, spirits of the plants used for healing, and spirits of animals. Shape shifting, the changing of one form into another, is sometimes included in their abilities. By exploring with open curiosity, anyone can begin to learn these things. As one develops and allows a deeper connection with the spirit world, they find their inner gifts and talents. By connecting to the medicine carried within, a shaman is able to cultivate their ability to sense, merge with and direct the life force of nature to regenerate what seems to be missing into a new, more holistic form. This is the law of abundance—ask and you shall receive.

Who Is a Kahuna?

In Hawaii, the term *kahuna* was traditionally used to describe a master of any craft such as a canoe builder, priest, navigator, or healer. A kahuna is one who can take powerful spiritual principles and apply them to the knowledge and skill of their craft to create impressive results. Although Hawaiians trained many kinds of kahuna for various purposes, they primarily used their keenly developed mind skills to effect change with intuitive knowledge of the laws of energy, compassion, and love—key components for their healing work's effectiveness.

One of our teachers, Uncle Harry, explains that the meaning of kahuna is better understood when treated as a verb rather than a noun. The energetic vibration of *kahuna* as a verb can be felt like a pulsating wave that moves through your body and affects different people in different ways. We have observed when working with people and their energetic matrices that healing actually takes place through a wave-form influence that carries a specific healing frequency. If one is recognized as a kahuna in their community, it is because they have dedicated themselves to following a tradition or preserving a legacy, and they have become adept at bringing about impressive results in their field of expertise. Thus kahuna science refers to consciously relating to the world in a way that brings everything around you into alignment. This is how a kahuna of "healing through prayer" could cure someone without even touching them, or how a kahuna of "prophesy" could see what would happen in the future and influence the coming events. In learning the art of lomi, we strive to apply these kahuna principles to healing the body at a soul level, creating permanent change.

2

Lomilomi— A Way of Life

*To gain the kingdom of heaven is to hear what
is not said, to see what cannot be seen, and
to know the unknowable—that is aloha.*
—Queen Lili'uakalani

People from all over the world make the journey to Hawaii looking to experience paradise. Hawaii is full of powerfully charged places to explore. When you visit the Hawaiian islands, you get a sense of something ancient beyond measure. Something begins to profoundly touch your soul. What creates this impact? When looking into the history of the place and its people, we discover stories that speak of power, passion, and miracles.

There are stories of amazing kahuna who could levitate large rocks, raise the dead, or alter the flow of lava from volcanoes. There are stories of working with the forces of nature to navigate across vast expanses of ocean. There are also stories of a mysterious and sacred connection to the stars, and these stories go beyond this realm of existence, involving the Sirius and Pleiades star systems, speaking of intergalactic travel. Woven through all the stories is a constant philosophy of stewardship. Nothing is more Hawaiian than the importance of understanding how people need to care for the earth, the ocean, and each other to nurture and co-maintain paradise as one united family.

A culture rooted in paradise is one that lives in a sacred and harmonious way, appreciating and honoring beauty, allowing an open heart and the voice of the earth to guide the way. All ancient cultures have roots in the creation of paradise reflected in their arts, spirituality, and heritage. Sometimes it may seem that our connection to paradise has been watered down or lost, and many of us have forgotten that our purpose is to bring heaven to this earthly plane. Yet in our own way, we all long to return to paradise. Our personal path to paradise is to express our soul's own unique way of creating something beautiful for others to enjoy. When we create beauty around us, we create paradise everywhere we go. In this way, we bring heaven to Earth.

Many who come to Hawaii begin to feel like they are in heaven, and this feeling of heaven is largely due to the isolated nature of the Hawaiian islands and the intensity of the elemental forces here. There is a particular quality of power that can be felt in the land, the ocean, the winds, and the forests. Located in the middle of the world's largest ocean, this small group of islands has always attracted adventurers from across the globe longing to discover its majestic secrets. Immersed in the beauty of Hawaii, you can begin to develop a relationship with the 'aina, the spirit of the land. And this is something that shifts and transforms you in a way that is hard to explain. For many who visit Hawaii, it is an experience that leaves them wanting more, a longing to somehow create that same feeling when they return home. This yearning leads many to explore the culture and the medicine of the Hawaiian people.

The vibrancy of the environment is reflected in the vibrancy of the people. When you spend time with the locals, participating and learning the ways of the culture, you begin to understand the deeper sense of strength that can be felt in the islands is largely because the Hawaiian people have taken care of their land in such a dedicated way. The strength of the Hawaiian people is reflected in the way they gather together to protect the environment, their families, and their way of life. Despite centuries of oppression, genocide, and the influences of the modern industries, many Hawaiian people have retained their way of caring for the land, the sea, and each other with reverence and respect—with aloha.

Aloha—A Way of Being

To effectively carry Hawaiian medicine, you must embody the spirit of aloha. Some of the deeper meanings of aloha have been preserved by a system of collective values, beginning with each letter of the word. These meanings offer guiding principles by which to live in harmony with each other, flowing through our actions, words, and deeds. This way of life is simply known as the way of aloha. (In the Hawaiian language, the *a* is pronounced as in "father." The *o* is pronounced as in "open." The *i* is pronounced as in "pita." The *e* is pronounced as in "prey." The *u* is pronounced as in "mood.")

- *Akahai*: careful offering, kindness, modesty, gentleness, tenderness, unpretentious, unassuming, unobtrusive

- *Lokahi*: obtain oneness, unity, agreement, accord, unison, harmony

- *Oluolu*: cool, refreshing, agreeable, pleasant, affability, amiability, contentment, happiness, graciousness, congeniality

- *Ha'ahaha*: humility, humbleness, self-effacing, modesty

- *Ahonui*: great breath, patience, perseverance, endurance, tolerance

Aloha means so much more than just hello or goodbye; it refers to the divine spirit of love that flows (as life) through all things. We have been taught aloha means "the breath of God is in our presence" and that it also means "I see the God in you." To say "aloha" acknowledges that the God that breathes life through you is the same God that breathes through all others. Many Hawaiians say that the only rule in saying aloha is to say it *only* when you really mean it. When you say aloha, it must come from your heart and soul. To say aloha when you do not truly mean it is a disgrace to its meaning and principle.

Hawaiian healing practices and the Hawaiian language have been growing in strength and popularity for many years now. In this age of information and communication, the teachings of the Hawaiian people have been set free in such a way that the brilliant light of aloha has spread far and wide. For many people involved in the healing arts, lomi is the primary way the message of aloha is conveyed through many cultures, as it is a great way to bring the teachings of aloha into action.

> *He kehau ho`oma`ema`e ke aloha*
> (Love is like a cleansing dew): The cleansing
> power of aloha can soothe and heal.

Hurt, pain, and suffering yield to aloha's healing power. By providing an experience of feeling deeply loved and nurtured, lomi regenerates us in every way, returning us to paradise. We find once again that place of comfort and wholeness, where we are free from guilt and fear. The masks and armor we wear in daily life can fall away, and we can have an experience of safety within unconditional love and support. True Hawaiian values teach us that aloha encompasses all people as equals and that we are all equally loved in every moment.

The teaching or practice of aloha is not limited by race, creed, age, sex, or style. The teachings of Hawaii are not to be restricted only to people of Hawaiian descent, but are to be shared and utilized by all who come with an open heart and a sincere dedication to living aloha and demonstrating a life of *pono*—righteousness. As North Americans teaching and giving lomi, we feel we have often been embraced by the Hawaiian people we have had the pleasure of connecting to, because they can feel that we strive to live, aloha. We have found that if you demonstrate a true respect for the land, have compassion for the struggles, and honor the culture, the people of Hawaii will embrace you and make you feel like part of their family.

You do not have to go to Hawaii to learn the healing methods that are inspired by the Hawaiian culture. There are many teachers all over the world who are on this path. But as you become more interested in the culture, you may wish to go there to become more rooted in the wisdom of the land and its people. In visiting Hawaii, you can connect to the land, get to know local people, and learn what you can from them. To fully understand Hawaiian healing, it is important to understand what it is to be Hawaiian and to understand how the aloha spirit works in all areas of life. Once this spirit is rooted within you, you can take it with you and bring the essence of aloha with you everywhere you go. When we are teaching, we feel the Hawaiian ancestors sharing their wisdom through us. In the true spirit of aloha, we also hold the wisdom and blessings of our own ancestors in equal esteem. We are honored to have developed a deeper connection to our ancestors as we continue to follow this path. We believe this is the wish of the Hawaiian ancestors: for the true meaning of aloha to be shared and shared by all, until it is commonly and universally understood and lived by all.

The Path of Pono

To be a giver of lomi, one learns to sustain a frequency of aloha by living in *pono*. Pono means goodness, harmony, and righteousness. To live in pono is to live for the greater good of the whole, taking care of ones-self, others, and the earth. This is why we look for good teachers, so that they can assist us not only with learning a healing technique, but also so that they can assist us to get back on track. *Kumu* means "instructor" as well as "source." So, a good lomi kumu is connected to the source of a particular lineage and will also show students how to connect to that divine source from within. Our teachers say it is not sufficient for us to have the *knowledge* of lomi; we must embody the spiritual principles, so that *wisdom* flows from within us and we can be a clear channel for spirit to work through us. A true teacher of lomi never considers themselves to be the one doing the healing—the spirit of aloha flows through us, offering healing to all.

In this time of rapid Earth changes, lomi has become invaluable because it can assist people today with the intense and often uncomfortable process of self-evolution; letting go of immature, old ways that no longer serve us, our families, or society. Healing is all about returning to a state of *pono*—living in right relationship. It is a way of life that involves deep feeling and attention to detail; a way of life that embraces all, accepts all and respects all.

It is understood that it is the prayers that actually cause the healing to take place, not the technique. The person coming to the table to receive a lomi is acknowledged as an innocent and sacred being worthy of unconditional acceptance, grace, and blessings. The lomi giver focuses on the perfection and wholeness of their receiver and bears witness to the immortality of their God-self, their eternal soul. This is the essence of lomilomi, and it is what keeps us all coming back for more.

Rooted deep in tradition, some practitioners still hold the space for the pure form of the traditional ways, and these selected individuals continue to practice the form, structure and protocol of specific traditional lineages of lomi. This is precious, as it holds the key to a wealth of ancient wisdom. These traditional practitioners can help connect us to the spirit of a people who hold all life as sacred. By learning from tradition, using prayers, chants, and protocols, we can awaken the part of ourselves that is ancient and sacred.

Styles of Lomi

Through perpetuating traditional practices of Hawaiian healing and spreading them throughout the world, the blessings and prayers of the ancestors are fulfilled. Some styles of lomi resemble those of ancient times. More modern styles can appear very different, having been adapted to serve the needs of the people today. All hold an intrinsic value. It is the purity of intention of the giver as well as the receiver, that when woven together creates an effective healing experience.

With its long, flowing, graceful strokes and deeply nurturing vibrations, Hawaiian massage has become so popular globally because it is such a comforting and heartfelt way of healing that will continue to thrive. The world needs an experience of healing that brings in prayer and gratitude and joy. Much of the lomi offered in spas and massage clinics has little resemblance to the traditional, tribal medicine ways, yet when practiced with sincerity of heart, it honors the spirit within. Though there are many styles of Hawaiian massage, these are the lineages shared in this book.

+ *Kahi Loa, the Touch of Magic*: Serge Kahili King

+ *Traditional Hawaiian Touch Medicine*:
  Harry Uhane Jim

+ *Big Island Lomi*: Aunty Margaret

+ *Heartworks, traditional Old Style lomi*:
  Sherman Dudoit

+ *Temple Style Lomi or Kahuna Bodywork*:
  Abraham Kawai'i

We introduce these lineages to give you an idea of the range of techniques involved when you hear the word *lomilomi*. All these styles of lomi are powerful and have great gifts to offer. We will aspire to convey the essence of the work, and later, we'll show you a few basic strokes and introduce you to the joint rotations. As you study different styles of lomi, you will eventually discover that there are common threads in all the styles. It is our desire to share these common threads with you. These are the ancient rhythms of spirit in motion.

3

The Physical

Lawe i ka ma'alea a ku'ono'ono—
Study and practice until it becomes a part of you

Lomilomi is the word given to many forms of healing bodywork treatments performed by the Hawaiian people. Here are just a few applications with their translations.

- *Lomi*: to knead, to squeeze, to break apart into smaller pieces

- *Lomilomi*: a soothing rub to relieve fatigue, limber up the muscle systems, and increase circulation

- *Ha'i ha'i*: a "breaking up" massage for when the body was full of kinks and the nervous system needed rebalancing

- *Ho'iho'i*: the replacement of organs that are out of position

+ *Ha'i ha'i iwi*: the Hawaiian practice of bone setting

+ *Manamana*: to heal another without touching

+ *Laulima*: the laying on of hands, by either one person or a group

+ *La'au lapa'au*: the use of plant medicines, considered an essential part of any lomi healing

Malama Ka 'Aina:
To Care for the Spirit of the Land

There is no way to authentically speak or write about Hawaiian spirituality unless you live it. The spiritual values and ceremonies of the Hawaiian people were woven into all the daily activities, such as fishing, paddling, harvesting medicines, or farming taro. To live it, you must have a balance between the spiritual and the material in all things in life. By having the right relationship with the land and all living things, we can be healthy, and we can have a healing effect on others. First is the concept of *malama ka 'aina*, care for the land and connection to the spirit of the land. There is nothing more Hawaiian than connecting intimately with your environment. This involves watching all the things going on around you, and seeing how they interact with each other, and with you. Indeed, *keiki* (children) were taught this at a very young age. They were trained how to communicate with the various aspects of nature by watching the sky, and attempting to move the clouds with their focused intention. The children learned skills by quietly watching their elders. By watching the elders or taking part in the daily activities such as farming taro, fishing, or surfing, important life lessons were learned.

He ali'i ka 'aina, he kauwa ke kanaka—
Land is the chief, people are its humble servants.

Kumu Anakala Pilipo Solatorio

For fifty generations, the family of Anakala Pilipo Solatorio has been farming taro in Halawa Valley, Molokai. We include him as one of our esteemed Hawaiian teachers because of all the cultural gifts he shared with us about Hawaiian protocols of an ancient way of life. Pilipo is a chanter and a kumu hula. He is known by many as a *kupuna*, an esteemed wise elder whose mastery lies in preserving the traditions and culture of the people of Molokai. He teaches us that in this life, all things are here for a reason and everything has purpose.

Uncle Pilipo also shares that it is up to each and every one of us to learn to live in pono with our surroundings and the people with whom we share our lives. If we desire to understand anything in life, there are plenty of signs all around us; we just have to pay attention! Uncle Pilipo offers up his traditional wisdom with an open heart to all who visit his home in Halawa Valley. He continues to demonstrate aloha, and share the ancient practices of protocol, hula, chant, weaving, taro farming, pounding poi, and the *mo'olelo* (stories) of the land of Halawa that were given to him by his ancestors.

By spending time in Halawa Valley with Uncle Pilipo and his 'ohana (family), we began to really slow down and witness how joining together in daily activities can be healing for the soul. By working with the land and the sea, we feed that part of ourselves which longs for a deeper connection to nature. In harvesting and preparing food as a family, we are nurtured and healed by the personal bonding we experience with the 'aina and each other.

EXERCISE: Blessing Your Property— Activating a Sacred Connection to Land

Preparation: This exercise takes place outside. You will be walking around the perimeter of your property, so dress with appropriate footwear, although barefoot is best. You can bring small gifts to place in the corners of the property or under certain trees or plants. These gifts could be water; small amounts of food; herbal offerings such as flowers, tobacco, or sage; specially selected crystals or stones; or other sacred decorations.

To begin: You can begin to malama ka 'aina (care for the spirit of the land) right here, right now, right where you live. Your home is your 'aina. The land you dwell on has a host of spirits, they are conscious and aware. The spirit of the land has a voice—honor it, for it is your friend. Begin by going outside and feeling your feet upon the ground. The ancestors' very life, blood, and bones are in the dirt beneath your feet.

Establish your sacred space by walking the perimeter of the property you live on. If you live in an apartment, you can do this in a nearby park or around your apartment building grounds. Give thanks to the trees and plants that line the perimeter, for they are your guardians. Observe all the plants on the property and feel how they support the area you live. Greet them with respect, touch the trees and feel their bark. Touch the plants and feel the leaves. Squeeze the leaves and smell their fragrance. Ask them to take care of you, as you care for them. Touch the soil, smell it, and run it through your fingers. Observe the way that the little creatures in and around the soil interact with the various plants on the land. There is an interdependent relationship between all life forms, and we can learn a lot from paying attention to these interactions.

Take a moment to acknowledge each living thing you come upon. *Ho'olohe mai!* Listen! What do you hear? Use your imagination. If they had voices, what would they be saying to you? If you pay attention, you can feel subtle differences in the breezes and see all the colors in the landscape. When you notice the beauty of creation, it takes on meaning. To malama ka 'aina is to love and to care for the spirit of each and every tree or tiny flower, every rock and every running stream and river.

As you walk the entire space of your property, ask if there is anything you can do to serve the spirits

there. Visit the trees that grow on the property and
thank them for being your protectors. Give them thanks
and offer water or perhaps a gift of food or a gift you
have prepared, such as a crystal or a sacred decora-
tion. If you see something that needs fixing, take the
time to beautify your surroundings—maybe trim
some bushes or clear some debris so that other plants
can thrive. After you are finished, take a moment and
breathe in and out as you stand upon your land and
feel grateful for the land and the home you have been
given. Your environment is a reflection of Creation's
love for you. Know as you listen to nature with the
ears of your heart that all of creation speaks. As you
speak, the ancestors hear you too. We are never alone.

La'au Lapa'au (Use of Plant Medicines)

Bodywork was just one part of Hawaiian healing. Each family
had healers who carried plant medicines and herbal formulas
to treat a variety of physical ailments. When offering healing,
the practitioner would carefully select plants to use, and herbal
treatments were incorporated with the massage. Hawaiians
understood plant medicine in its many applications such as
poultices, oils, ointments, herbal or salt rubs, colon cleansers,
tonics, and teas. The practitioner would call first to the spirits
and then listen carefully to determine which plant wanted to
assist that particular person in their healing. There were specific chants used for calling to the gods and goddesses. These

protocols and chants were used for going into the forest to look for the plant that wanted to help the person who was coming for healing. Finding the right plant was a very intuitive process, and the method was a key aspect of Hawaiian healing, much the same as practices in other indigenous cultures that use plant medicine for healing.

In his book *Plant Spirit Medicine*, Eliot Cowan says that an effective practitioner must develop a personal way of connecting to and calling in the spirit of a plant. The spirit comes in and delivers the perfect type of blessing for the person using it. He writes:

> Plant Spirit Medicine is a macro-religious rite in which plant gods bestow their grace. How is that grace invoked? Some people use song, others use pills or potions, still others lay on hands, wave feathers, or dance. Who knows how many ways are waiting to be discovered or rediscovered? Whatever method is used, the spirits are invited to help the patient enter the dream of nature; this has nothing to do with fighting illness. For us, there is no such thing as an herb that is good for arthritis or migraine or depression or cancer. Whatever medicine a plant gives you, that's what it will do for your patients … If you want to use a plant for healing, you have to dream it, or it won't work for you … Rarely do two people have exactly the same dreams. Rarely do two people use the same plant in exactly the same way.

Begin by looking at the plants that grow naturally in the area where you live. Work with any plant that calls to you, and develop a close relationship with it. Research its properties and medicinal uses. Plants that grow wild in the natural settings in which you live offer the perfect vibrational medicine to help you through whatever you are experiencing. It is said by some medicine people that nature does not create an illness that she does not provide a cure for, and the cure is always growing in the area where the illness appears. By researching the local plant life, you can learn to use herbs and discover which ones work best for you.

The medicinal plants used in Hawaii are a joy to explore. If you are interested in becoming a practitioner of Hawaiian medicine, it is a good idea to get to know some of the plants used in Hawaii and develop a relationship with their medicinal properties. Here are just a few of the most common and accessible plants used by the people of Hawaii today.

Hawaiian Plant Medicines

Kukui nut: The kukui tree is very important to the people of
   Hawaii because of its oil, which was used to light torches
   for night fishing and lamps. Because of its use as a source
   of light, it is spiritually associated with bringing light into
   your being. The kukui nuts are worn as a lei around the
   neck for this purpose. The nut is also edible. Eaten raw it
   is a powerful laxative, and when roasted it becomes a tasty
   condiment. The kukui nut oil was used for massage and

was also rubbed on the body for spiritual protection, or protection from the sun. In lomilomi, the nut of the kukui tree was crushed and applied to the limbs of the body as a rub or warmed and used as a poultice.

Awa: Commonly called kava or kavakava, Awa is used widely among Islanders throughout the Pacific. Many cultures drink Kava recreationally, enjoying the sense of relaxation it brings. In Hawaii, it is a sacred offering to the ancestors. The roots of the Awa plant are dried, crushed into a powder, and then made into a beverage. This beverage is drunk in a ceremonial fashion. It is used as a spiritual medicine, to unite a group together for a process such as ho'oponopono or connecting to the ancestors. Medicinally, it was used by paddlers and in childbirth because it could help to relax tired, aching muscles.

Noni: This tree is highly regarded by the people of the Polynesia as a life-giving or even lifesaving plant. It grows in abundance in the islands and can easily be spotted by its stinky yellow fruit that falls to the ground when ripe. Noni leaves are applied directly to the body for pain relief for bruises, sprains, sore muscles, or to soothe the breasts of a breast-feeding mother. Noni fruit can be eaten raw or specially made into a juice, and it is also used internally for a variety of ailments such as a tonic to boost the immune system.

'Olena: Commonly called turmeric, 'olena was used internally and externally to cleanse, strengthen, relieve inflammation and purify the body. Sprinkling turmeric-infused saltwater in the corners of a room was thought to dispel negative energy or spirits.

Ti: The ti plant is a very sacred plant to the Hawaiian people and can be seen growing all over Hawaii. It was used for many things, such as: leis worn for protection and purification, wrapping sacred offerings for the altar, and also wrapping fish or vegetables for cooking. The ti plant was planted near burial plots in ancient times, and the spirits of the ancestors buried in these plots fortified the ti plant with mana. Today, the ti leaf is commonly planted in the four corners of one's property and by the entrance of one's home for protection and blessing of the home. In lomilomi, a ti leaf could be used to bless the person, used to sprinkle saltwater on the person, and bless the space the healing was taking place in to bring protection into the healing space. The ti leaf was also used to wrap a *pohaku* (stone), then placed on the body for use as a hot pack to relax the muscles. The ti leaf is very soothing when applied directly to the body for headaches or other types of pain relief, and the juice or root of the plant was used for healing cuts and wounds.

Alaea: Alaea is a type of red clay gathered from specific locations on the Hawaiian islands that is very high in iron oxide. The clay was traditionally fed to patients as a supplement for its mineral content and nutritional value. Salt gathered from sea water was mixed with alaea and baked, creating alaea salt, also known as Hawaiian salt. This salt was and still is used for cooking and for healing. Alaea salt was considered very sacred because the clay is symbolic of the connection to the ancestors. It is considered a sacred offering, that is also used as a gift to show proper respect to a kahuna or kupuna. The kahuna used water mixed with alaea to cleanse and bless people or objects, and it was sprinkled around the home to purify the energy in the home and please the ancestors. Alaea salt is used in lomilomi as a stimulating, exfoliating rub for the skin. A bowl of alaea salt is often used under the table in a lomi session to gather and extract negative energy from the body.

Kai: Sea water: Colon cleansing was an essential part of Hawaiian Healing practices. Pure sea water from the deep ocean was commonly used for a colon cleanser. This was usually done by fasting for a few days and then drinking the sea water to flush the elimination system.

Ha: The Breath of Life

Ha is the breath of life that contains the energy of our Creator. Because it was the creator who breathed into us to give us life, our breath is always our connecting chord back to the source. We are given Ha (our breath) to have a constant reminder that the Divine is living in us, breathing through us, as us, and for us. Any time we desire to hear the voice of God, we breathe and listen from deep within. To hear the quiet voice of our higher self, we must quiet the chatter in our mind. This is most readily achieved by focusing on one's breathing. For Hawaiians, the concept of Ha is simple—if you don't breathe, you die!

The Ha breath is a powerful and efficient healing tool that allows stuck emotional energy to surface and be transmuted into light. It is also used in healing to infuse the cells of the body with mana (power). By breathing along with someone else, you make a direct connection to their whole being. The breath opens you up to sense the presence of the ancestors and helpful spirits or angels. You can assist another to heal by breathing into any part of their body that needs healing. You can use your own breath to "pull out" or extract unwanted energies from their body.

In the context of a bodywork session, different breathing patterns create different frequencies, all of which affect the physical body. A general rule of thumb for any style of bodywork is to pay attention to the breathing pattern of your receiver. Deep pressure strokes are applied on their exhalation and lightened as they begin to inhale. You may notice at times the client breathing very deeply or breathing in a constricted way. These indications show you where energy is blocked in their body, which can be released on their exhale. In those places of constriction, extra attention, sensitivity, and focus are required to open the energy in those areas. By encouraging them to deepen their breathing, more light will flow in, dissolving the blockage.

EXERCISE: The Ha Breathing Technique

Breathe in deeply, beginning from the belly. Raise the breath up into the heart and exhale with a "haaah" sound—this is Ha breathing. This simple exercise can transform your whole day. Ha breathing was done before any chant, prayer, or ceremonial activity in Hawaii to build up *mana* (life force energy) and create an opening to the higher self.

Preparation: This exercise can be done seated anywhere at any time. Do the exercise for a short period of time (one to five minutes) to balance, clear, and energize yourself throughout the day. It can also be done lying down for a longer period of time (five to twenty minutes) for deeper healing effects such as releasing emotions or stuck energy. You can do this seated or lying comfortably in your bed.

To begin: Move your body around a bit to loosen up, and begin to straighten out your spine in whatever position you are in; standing, sitting, or lying down. Relax your jaw and inhale through the mouth. Breathing from your belly, let it relax and expand. Raise the breath up into the top of your lungs, expanding the chest and heart area. Exhale slowly through the mouth, with a "Haaah" sound. Repeat for several minutes and notice any sensations in your body as you keep breathing.

The Training of a Lomi Practitioner

In traditional times, the first thing a student was taught was how to live in pono. They learned to address any imbalance in themselves and their relationships before working on another. In their training, they learned specific chants and prayers to honor the gods, goddesses, and ancestor spirits. They learned about all the common illnesses; how to diagnose them in the body by running their hands over the body; and how to gather, bless, and apply herbs for these illnesses. Then they were ready to be taught the art of lomilomi massage and bodywork. Much of the bodywork was learned from watching the kahuna do the work, as mentioned earlier. Students in old Hawaii were taught to be very alert and pay attention to what the teacher was doing, and also to remain quiet and wait before asking questions. This encouraged the student to discover the answer on their own, rather than being given information they were not ready to understand.

Haha: To Diagnose Through One's Hands

A lomi student was traditionally taught to run their hands over the body of the person receiving treatment to sense the energetic field and to diagnose the probable cause of the ailment. To train in the practice of Haha, the student was given a bucket of pebbles that were carefully chosen. When all were laid out, the pebbles would form the shape of a human body. Each pebble had a specific place. The student had to memorize each pebble and its position in the layout of the body. Each position of each pebble had significance, and with practice the student was able to locate specific pebbles with eyes closed by running their hands over the layout. The student was taught how different ailments in the body correlate to different parts of the stomach. In this way, the student was taught about how to feel or scan for various illnesses and where they are located in the body. Traditionally, the student of Hawaiian healing was not introduced to massage or bodywork techniques until they learned many other protocols.

EXERCISE: Scanning the Body with Hands

Preparation: This exercise can be done on yourself, a pet, or a friend. If you are alone, you can sit on the floor or in a chair and just run your hands over your own body. If you are with someone else, you can have them lie on the floor or a massage table, or they can sit in a chair in front of you.

To begin: Place your hands over the body of your receiver or over your own body. You can begin at the head area and move down the body. Once you get to the feet, you can go back up the body again if you wish, and finish at the head area again.

Hold your hands a few inches away from the body, and see if you can feel the energy field. Move away slowly, and then move in closer again. You should be able to detect an energetic layer between two to four inches away from the body. Begin to move slowly over the body with your eyes closed, and feel the differences in the energy as you move along. Move slowly and notice if you feel pulled to a certain place more strongly than another.

As you slowly move down the body and explore every area, notice the differences in the energy as you go. Do you feel places that are warmer or colder? Do you feel places that are prickly or smooth? Some places may feel like a hole that needs filling, or there may be energy that feels built up that wants to be released. You can share with the person you are scanning what you are sensing and see if they feel anything there too. You can also see if any messages or images come to you as you listen and feel through your hands. Perhaps you will be surprised at what you receive.

4

The Spiritual

Hawaiian healing works through connecting with the divine—the spirit that dwells within us and in all things. This involves calling to various spirit allies for assistance, and it also works through addressing the ancestral wounds on a personal soul level. We will address each of these aspects, beginning with the teachings of the three souls or three aspects of self. Following is Serge King's explanation of this system to lay some foundations:

"The concept of three selves in Hawaiian culture is not traditional in the sense that it is common throughout the culture. It is an esoteric tradition taught by some families. Max Freedom Long created an esoteric system based on his interpretation of Hawaiian words and certain Theosophical ideas. For a long time there wasn't much else available, so some Hawaiians adopted his system and others rejected it. I was taught the esoteric system of the Kahili family and was the first of that lineage to make it public in the seventies. Long's idea was that we are all composed of three spirits, two of which reside in the body and the other floats above it. One he called the lower self and he used the word 'unihipili—defined in 1865 as a graduated animal spirit that has been reborn into a human body. Next in Long's system is the middle self, a lower self spirit that has graduated to a higher level. For this he used the word 'uhane, defined in 1865 as the spirit of a deceased person and also used by the missionaries as a translation for soul. Long decided that this was the word for the spirit that forms our conscious mind. For naming the higher self he picked the word 'aumakua, a good choice since it was used by Hawaiians to represent ancestral spirits and also the word for someone whose ordinary spirit could be purposely transformed into a guardian spirit. For Long, though, this was a graduated middle self that hovered above and provided energy (defined as *mana* by Long) to the middle self when requested through the lower self."

Dr. King continues: "My uncle Wana Kahili taught that everything is spirit, whether focused into form (*kino*) or not. *Ku* is the term used for the physical (body) spirit—meaning to exist, anchor, to stand, to appear, and was a god of natural things like fish and fishing, hunting, gathering, and so on. Lono is used for the mental spirit, or mind—meaning of news, to listen, to be attentive and it was a god of more intellectual things like medicine, agriculture, and navigation. *Kane* is used for what we also call the higher self, but which is more like an oversoul that transcends time and space. This comes from a root meaning of *ka-ane*, the breath of life, and was the god of mountaintops and rain from the heavens. Originally it was *kanewahine*, reflecting the dual or androgynous nature of this aspect. These spirits are not separate, but spiritual aspects of one being and represent the functions of memory, imagination, and inspiration, respectively."

With the above in mind, it is important to note that lomilomi is a vehicle for the alignment of body, mind, and spirit. These three aspects of our being are known to have their own individual soul consciousness and were acknowledged for their own unique contributions to the whole. To understand, integrate, and harmonize these three souls is essential to one's well-being. To know how to communicate with each one of our souls helps us understand the healing process. We combine what we have learned from our various teachers:

- *Ku ('Unihipili, Subconscious, Body, Child)*: Hawaiians often refer to the *'unihipili* as "the soul that clings." This is because it is a soul that is inhabiting (clinging to) our body during our earthly incarnation. We use our body to communicate energetically with the world around us, sending and receiving communication through the *aka*, energetic connections. The body is constantly taking in information and processing the commands of both the conscious mind (*lono*) and the higher self (*kane*). It listens, processes, records, and then speaks to us through symbols and sensations in the body as well as through our emotions. Hawaiian teachings tell us that when we want something, our mind sends a command to the *ku* (the child), which will begin to generate an energetic pattern of attraction and gather all the ingredients to fulfill the desired outcome.

This self was referred to as the child, because of the way that it is always drawn toward pleasure. Our ku loves pleasing tastes, smells, sounds, sights, and feelings, and it will always be attracted to energies and sensations it finds entertaining and enjoyable. Ku is the consciousness of the body and the storehouse of our memory. It remembers every thought the mind tells it, and it stores the memory of all events in our body. The body attaches feelings to the memories, and when a memory is triggered, the body sends that feeling to the mind again for the purpose of communication. It will do its best to steer us away from anything that will cause us any pain or discomfort. Much like a child, the ku needs training to be guided away from unhealthy or destructive associations and behaviors. The process of repatterning the body and mind works best when using repetition and reward … much like training a dog.

As ku is directly connected with kane; the body can be used to receive clear guidance from our higher self. This makes ku a receiver of great power and wisdom. Divine guidance is communicated through our body in the form of physical sensations, like goose bumps, tingles, emotional or intuitive feelings, or sudden cramps. The messages and impulses we receive from ku are felt in our *na'au* (gut). If our body is sending us a positive feeling, this means that our thoughts are in alignment with our higher wisdom. If we are getting a bad feeling from our body, it is telling us that our thoughts are out of alignment with our divine wisdom and something needs to be adjusted. Lomilomi is a unique form of healing due to how it honors the body as a source of divine energy and wisdom, enabling us to connect with infinity. Because it stores our memory, our body needs to align its energy for healing to take place. When it feels safe and loved, it will gladly open and release trauma, wounds, and stuck energy from the body.

+ *Lono ('Uhane, Mind, Conscious Awareness, Parent):* Hawaiians often refer to *'uhane* as "the soul that talks." This is because this is the part of us that is always thinking and speaking in words. 'Uhane or *lono*, the spirit of our will, has the ability to direct our attention, make decisions, and give commands to our ku. Our lono is the part of us that creates through thoughts, words, and focused attention. Because it stores our memory, our body is required to align its energy with the divinity within it for healing to take place. When it feels acknowledged, safe, and loved, it will then soften and allow the release of trauma, unforgiven wounds, and stuck energy. To do this, we must pause, think, take a breath, and speak slowly. This gives us time to let our feelings catch up with our minds and the higher self to guide our words appropriately.

Take a moment to think about how you move throughout your daily life. Do your words match your feelings? Do your words match your heart's desires? The true purpose of our mind is to function as a humble servant to the higher self, focused on the greatest good with the heart and the mind united. Our 'uhane creates volition toward our creativity while using our imagination and determination. Used properly, it can help us engage and fulfill our life purpose on Earth. In a lomilomi session, the practitioner, in cooperation with the person receiving treatment, uses their 'uhane to focus on an image or a thought that creates healing vibrations. The best thing a lomilomi practitioner can learn to do is to quiet their mind, bring their focus into the present moment, and mentally call to their higher self ('aumakua), to come forward and work lovingly with their body's intuitive wisdom (our unihiplili) to create a pathway for positive change.

* Kane (Higher Self, Super Conscious, 'Aumakua, Spirit, Oversoul, God Self): The concept of 'Aumakua relates to one's ancestors. But in the huna system it refers to the oversoul, or higher self. To understand this concept, it

is important to note that the Hawaiian language is not a language of separation. The Hawaiian culture is not based on duality; it is based on *lokahi* (unity). And so the word 'Aumakua refers to the union of your higher self along with the higher selves of your whole family lineage; past, present, and future.

Hale Makua, the kahuna featured in the book, *The Bowl of Light* by Hank Wesselman describes the 'Aumakua. "The ancestors, including our own personal creative principle, our 'Aumakua, higher oversoul, or as some would say our God Self, exists on a sub-level above us on which we come to discover that each of us belongs to a family of souls. These are oversouls that have frequent and ongoing contact with each other as we journey toward the future. And they, in turn, are members of the ancestral group soul matrix, *Ka Po'e 'Aumakua*, the great gathering of human oversouls. This is what people call the human spirit, although most of us who use this term do not understand what it really means."

Kahuna Hale Makua says that when we breathe our last breath, all of our earthly experience—the lessons and love attained throughout our human journey—is breathed back into our 'aumakua's matrix of light to be digested, nurturing its growth and evolution. Your 'aumakua was here long before you came into this body, and it will be here long after you die. It is anchored in Truth, knowing your destiny, purpose, and your heart's desire. This is the witness aspect of you, which is in connection to all your guides and ancestors. It can access all times and dimensions. This part of your consciousness is the creator aspect. It's connected to the realm of the un-manifest, where it can access and harness higher vibrational frequencies to create reality in the physical dimension.

Much like angels or spirit guides, our higher self has a subtle way of working in our lives and can be felt and used most effectively when it is consciously invited. It knows all and sees all but does not interfere with your choices and lacks the capacity to judge. Occasionally, it might intrude upon a situation to save us from an untimely death or dangerous events that do not serve us. Used properly, our higher self can be a constant comforter and companion, guiding us and feeding us energy and inspiration from the upper realms for our creative projects. With practice, your higher self can connect you to all things through the *aka* web, allowing you visions, psychic messages, astral travel, and intuitive sensations all received through your body. By keeping in close communication with the 'aumakua, we can call for help when we need it. This can be a life saver when you are really struggling. By understanding the connection of the 'aumakua, you can work with all your guides, guardians, and ancestors to make great things happen in your life. In a lomi session, it is considered helpful for the person needing healing to appeal to their own 'aumakua for assistance through prayer offerings and the intentional use of Ha breathing.

Eight Principles of Hawaiian Healing

We love what we are able to invite into life through practicing Dr. King's teachings, Ka Ike Huna in particular. He has written several books where he clearly outlines what he calls the seven principles of huna. (In the Hawaiian language, the *a* is pronounced as in "father." The *o* is pronounced as in "open." The *i* is pronounced as in "pita." The *e* is pronounced as in "prey." The *u* is pronounced as in "mood.")

- *Ike*: Awareness: The world is what you think it is

- *Kala*: Freedom: There are no limits

- *Makia*: Focus: Energy flows where attention goes

- *Manawa*: Presence: Now is the Moment of Power

- *Aloha*: Love: To love is to be happy

- *Mana*: Power: All power comes from within

- *Pono*: Goodness: Effectiveness is the measure of truth

For our *halau* (school), Kealohi added an eighth principle, *Malu* (peace), to remind us that all the other principles can lead us back to a profound peacefulness within our human experience. Aunty Mahealani, a wise kupuna, was so kind to assist Kealohi in sharing her Hawaiian proverbs that best suited each of the principles from Dr. King. Through her many gifts, she brings a feminine balance and integrity to this esoteric from the Kahili clan. Aunty is truly the embodiment of a pure Hawaiian heart—we thank her for all the great work she does in the world to preserve the Hawaiian culture and honor the way of aloha.

Hawaiian Proverbs for Healing

+ Ike: *Ike moakaaka o keiki maka*: I see clearly through the eyes of a child

+ Kala: *Noa mai pilikia*: I am free from trouble of any kind

+ Makia: *Eia*: I am here

+ Manawa: *Ola manawa ike manawa*: I live moment to moment

+ Aloha: *Pu'u wai hamama*: My heart space is open

+ Mana: *Ikaika*: I stand in my power

+ Pono: *Aloha 'Uhane*: I greet with love the greatness of my Spirit

+ Malu: *'Uawo:* I create peace

Hawaiian Principles for Healing

+ Ike (Awareness) *Ike, moakaaka, o keiki maka*: I see clearly through the eyes of a child. When you see

things without judgment, you can see them in innocence. Awareness is all there is; being aware of itself.
All energy is self-aware, just being itself. Everything
around you is responding to your awareness. *Key:* All
things mean *only* what they mean to you.

+ Kala (Freedom) *Noa mai pilikia:* I am free of trouble;
  released from all ties that bind me to a story that has
  expired. Live in your truth, yet allow others to have
  their truth, and be themselves, loving one another.
  Key: Be in love with letting go!

+ Makia (Focus) *Eia:* I am here; focused within (my)
  authentic presence, merging with, or influencing
  the 'current,' of energy, and manifesting my reality
  through the gravity of focused attention. *Key:* Be
  aware of what you are focusing on, as it will multiply.

+ Manawa (Presence) *Ola manawa ike manawa:* I live
  moment to moment. There is only now! No other
  moment actually exists. It is only in this moment that
  my 'presence' lives and thrives. *Key:* Be here now.

+ Aloha (Love) *Pu'u wai hamama:* My heart space is
  open. Only love is immortal. Nothing immortal can
  be threatened. Pure love accepts all things, embraces
  all things, transcends all things! *Key:* Always follow
  the gravity of love.

+ Mana (Power) *Ikaika*: I stand strong in my power.
Spiritual authority comes from within. Personal
confidence directs a bounty of treasures revealed
through a true warrior's humility. *Key:* Know and live
the strength of impeccable devotion to the integrity
of love, generated from within a humble, surrendered
heart.

+ Pono (Goodness) *Aloha 'Uhane*: I greet with love the
greatness of my spirit. The goodness of our spirit can
flow when we walk a righteous path. *Key:* Effectiveness emerges through flexibility; aspire to be in right
relationship within yourself, within the world, and
within all your relations.

+ *Malu (Peace) 'Uawo*: I create peace, serenity, safety.
True peace is accessible to the one who allows everything to be, just as it is. *Key:* Be still, humble, respectful, honoring infinite grace, fully present, aware, and
trusting of divine right order.

Here are phrases of the main qualities imbedded in these
Hawaiian words. You may use the affirmations for chanting to
open and enhance the energy field within and around you.

+ *Ike, Kala, Makia, Manawa, Aloha, Mana, Pono, Malu*

+ I Am Aware, I Am Free, I Am Here, I Am Present

+ I Am Love, I Am Strong, I Am Good, I Am Peace

Pule (Prayer)

All healing is generated from a higher level than the physical level, where the disease is showing up. So it's always wise to summon help from the spirit realms above and within to effect a healing. It is the role of a lomi giver to become a vessel for the power of spirit to work through them. A *haumana* (student) of lomilomi in pre-Christian times was taught many different prayers, chants, and protocols for calling in the ancestors, gods, and goddesses to assisting a healing. When Christianity was adopted into the Hawaiian culture, their prayers began to change form. The complex protocols and ceremonies of the past were simplified, and many Hawaiian healers incorporated Bible verses and prayers to Jesus into their practice. To this day, prayer performed with reverence, love, and sincerity is still considered the main ingredient of any lomi healing. We encourage you to practice praying in your own way, as often as possible. We share here many different aspects of prayer, and provide examples of how prayer can be woven into your own personal healing as well as your private practice.

Oli (Chant)

There is nothing quite like the sound of a Hawaiian chant. It is a unique form of chanting that carries the richness and wisdom of the ancient culture. The reciting of chants was used for communication, called in the various gods and goddess, and united people while performing a task. It was how each family lineage preserved their ancestral history and legacy. The dance known as *hula* (sacred dance) was used in combination with chant to help to convey and remember the legends and stories, and send messages to the people or to the gods and goddesses. Chanting was often used to begin a lomi session to raise the vibration of both giver and receiver, and to open to the blessing and assistance of the ancestors, inviting the Halau guardians and ke akua to assist.

Upon the arrival of the missionaries, chanting and hula were banned in Hawaii. Many of the chants of the *kanaka maoli* (native Hawaiian) were buried or lost. To study the remaining traditional chants is one of the only ways to access what is left of a great cultural treasure. After they were forced into the shadows, the chants were used to convey an important message to a specific group of people and often contained a hidden meaning, a *kauna*, so that only certain people understood. Learning hula is a wonderful way to learn the stories and chants of the people of Hawaii as well as live and experience the living spirit of aloha. You can use the Hawaiian proverbs provided in this book, and we also provide more short Hawaiian chants you can try in later chapters. You may also enjoy the adventure of creating your own chants in your own language.

'Ohana (Family)

Family and food are very important aspects of Hawaiian life. Without strong, united families, a tribe cannot endure. Tribal peoples had many children so their lineage could grow, and of course without adequate food both physical and spiritual, the 'ohana could not be healthy and strong. In ancient times, before the Tahitians introduced the ali'i (royalty) hierarchical system based upon exclusion and rules, Hawaiian society was run by the 'ohana system of sustainability and peaceful coexistence. The concept of 'ohana applies to all aspects of life and spirituality. Note the smaller word *ha* in the middle of 'o-ha-na. This indicates the sharing of the Ha (breath) between family members as being the origin of life. This is symbolized by a greeting called *honi*. The honi is usually used in Pacific Island cultures between family and close friends or other respected acquaintances. It is done by two people coming forehead to forehead to share a Ha breath with eyes closed or open, connecting soul to soul with deep reverence. The greeting is also commonly done by touching one's cheek to another's cheek.

'Ohana and Lomilomi

In Hawaii, the concept of family relations extends to all life— including plants, animals, and the elements. You become connected by observing nature closely and how everything interacts together and with you personally. This intimate connection enables you to draw upon powerful mana, harnessing the fortitude of nature, to facilitate a healing. The entire family is connected through the aka, including those who have passed and those yet to be born. Lomilomi promotes the healing of all our family relations and facilitates the maturation of ancestral patterns by releasing the energetic ties which are holding the patterns in place. In this way, our personal healing affects our whole family—past, present, and future.

The concept of 'ohana was used to understand all relationships. This extends into thoughts and beliefs. Kahu Abraham Kawai'i referred to these as "food for the family," and beliefs as members of the "family of beliefs." Every thought carries energy—food for the family—such as fear, love, anger, and joy. So we must examine what we are feeding our family and which member of the family we are feeding. If you want less drama, don't feed the family of drama! If we want more joy, we feed the family of joy.

Abraham had a saying, that "the good, the bad, and the ugly are all family." We want to embrace all feelings, just as we embrace all family members. The way of aloha is inclusive; it does not encourage the rejection of any family member, because everyone has value and deserves to have a say. It is healthier to integrate the parts of ourselves or other people who challenge us in life than it is to cast them out. By accepting these uncomfortable vibrations, they become family and can empower us and enrich the understanding of our own shadow nature. On this, Kahu said, "When you approach something or someone as family, it will become family."

'Ohana Soulmate Systems

Each time we incarnate, we may choose a different character in our birth-family lineage to play. This is how the soulmate system of your birth family operates on Earth—through interactive, integrated soul recycling. Maybe you played the father this time and the mother last time. A grandparent may return to you as your child, so that they can stay close to you. Each life-time, as souls progress through earthly incarnations, we learn to love each other from a different role and evolve our own soul through playing all the unique roles in a given family lineage, or soulmate system. This of course extends beyond the family bloodline. Often we encounter others we have known in previous lifetimes and together we work out our unresolved issues that began in a previous life.

Three Circles of Relationship

Uncle Harry teaches the concept of three primary circles of relationship:

+ *First ring*: Your primary relationship with yourself; the inner circle that includes the inner 'ohana of your soul cluster—your body, mind, and spirit.

+ *Second ring*: Your relationship with your immediate family members, the ones you actually live with and relate to every day, which would include your spouse, lover, partner, parents, children, and pets.

+ *Third ring*: Your relationship with extended 'ohana: your casual acquaintances, community, and the world at large.

Think of these as three circles within each other: inner, middle, and outer. All relationship patterns begin within our inner cir-cle, forming ripples that extend outward. If we want to improve our relationships with our family members or the world at large, we must first strengthen and harmonize the relationships within our first, inner circle—our body, mind, and spirit: *ku*, *lono*, and *kane*.

Na 'Aumakua (The Ancestors)

Our family lineage evolves harmoniously when we *malama pono* (take care of things with integrity) on our personal journey on Earth. We would not be where we are today without the many challenges our ancestors faced. If it wasn't for them, we would not be alive today, and so we must always remember to honor our ancestors for the many gifts they have brought us. In the opening prayers of any type of gathering or ceremony in Hawaii, the presence of the ancestors is always acknowledged and blessed. The ancestors from the family lineage who had great personal power and achieved wondrous things in life were looked upon as akua (gods and goddesses), such as Pele, Lono, and Maui. These powerful ascended beings were honored in prayers, chants, and hula, and revered as protectors and guides for all people.

In ancient Hawaii, the spirits of ancestral guardians were believed to have the ability to shapeshift and move through space and time, taking on many different forms such as animals, rocks, rainbows, or thunder to communicate and announce their presence. Hawaiian families associate a specific animal with their 'aumakua (ancestors) such as the shark, owl, turtle, and so on. Each of us carries talents that were passed on to us from our ancestors, and it is our responsibility to develop these gifts and take them to the next level. If we are using the gifts to live our lives in a good way, then we are feeding our ancestors with our mana; in return, they give us more of their mana and assistance. For this reason, we have nearly limitless energy when we do something we really love. It may displease your ancestors to deny your talents, and doing so may cause them to withdraw their energy and support. When we do not have our ancestors' support, it can leave us feeling uninspired, empty, and eventually make us ill.

There are many sacred sites where temples were placed for specific purposes. These areas are *kapu*, closed off to tourists, for they act as an energetic container for all the prayers of those who have gone before. Powerful ancestral guardians still continue to inhabit these sites, and permission before entering is required. Much care is taken not to offend the ancestors in thought, word, or deed, for it is believed by many that this is the cause of misfortune or disaster. Many people tell stories of encounters with ghosts in Hawaii, such as the ones known as the night marchers, the spirits of ancient warriors.

When approaching a location of great power, such as a *heiau* (temple), it is important to ask permission from the ancestors to enter by saying *E kala mai*, which means "excuse me," or "please clear (or open) the way, I am coming through." You wait for a sign from nature to indicate if there is some reason not to enter. If you saw a big branch or a rock fall, that would likely be a sign to not enter. But if the reply was a welcoming song of a bird or sweet warm Hawaiian breeze blowing into the heiau, the indication would be that you are welcome and it is safe to enter.

Lomilomi and na 'Aumakua

In traditional lomi teachings, illness is caused by incorrect thoughts, words, and deeds. In our blood, we carry the wisdom as well as the unresolved issues of our ancestors. In this way, the issues of our ancestors may become our issues today. The act of lomilomi helps release the memories of these patterns, evolving our being on the level of our DNA. As we heal, the spirits of our ancestors also heal and evolve along with us. It is also believed that through our choices, when our descendants (grandchildren, great-grandchildren, etc.) are ready to join us here in this dimension, they come in with a higher level of consciousness, and with less baggage to process in their new lives.

By replacing destructive patterns with more harmonious ones, we teach other members of our family by example. Doing so evolves the entire family bloodline. In lomilomi we intend to clear the past and future generations within *pa'a* (the present). If there was conflict between the men and the women in our families before, there is usually an imbalance within our own inner masculine and feminine energies. The healing between the masculine and feminine within us can be extremely powerful work, especially when done in connection to the ancestors within the family lineage.

We begin every lomi session by calling in, acknowledging, and thanking the ancestors for their blessings. We call to both the paternal and maternal bloodlines, and tune in to the oversoul matrix of the 'aumakua. We can often feel lingering disharmony between the men and the women of the family going back generations and encourage forgiveness. In persons of mixed bloodlines, we often sense the judgments these ancestors have for each other based on cultural conditioning. We ask them to let go of their judgments for each other. The asking does not have to be verbalized, but doing these things with the conscious participation of the client is very potent, so that they can deepen their relationships with their 'aumakua. By using their breath, a strong intention, and a guided forgiveness process, one can clear the way for more harmony in the whole family lineage—a huge blessing and healing for all.

Ho'oponopono (To Make Right, Conflict Resolution)

A big part of life in old Hawaii was *ho'oponopono*—the practice of forgiveness and conflict resolution that brings order and harmony to your inner being and your external relationships. Ho'oponopono must be taken care of first to clear the path for any illness or tension to leave the body. It involves a recognition and expression of your deepest feelings, followed by a release of energetic ties and a resolution through grace. The Hawaiian word for this release is *kala*—to untie the knot, to free, to unbind. When we harbor judgments, all our energy gets tied up in knots, causing too much tension and sometimes illness in the body. Forgiveness is the primary tool used to untie the knots.

The traditional ho'oponopono process was facilitated through ceremony. The whole family would gather when grievances needed to be settled. In serious cases, an elder would preside. For everyday-type issues, there was also the 'ohana process of ho'oponopono, which involved the family sitting in a circle before bedtime, going one by one around the circle so that each member of the family could clear away any negative energy before going into dreamtime. This kind of ho'oponopono was also done by some individuals at the end of the day in quiet contemplation and prayer, and it was taught to the children at a very young age through the parable "A Bowl of Perfect Light," an ancient Hawaiian story. The following is a version from *Tales from the Night Rainbow* by Pali Jai Lee and Koko Willis:

A Bowl of Perfect Light

Each child has, at birth, a bowl of perfect light. If he tends to his light, it will grow in strength and he can do all things— swim with sharks, fly with the birds, know and understand all things. If however he becomes envious, jealous, angry, or fearful, he drops a stone into his bowl of light and some of the light goes out. Light and the stone cannot hold the same space. If he continues to put stones in the bowl, the light will go out and he will become a stone himself. A stone does not grow, nor does it move. If at any time he tires of being a stone, all he needs to do is turn the bowl upside down and the stones will fall away and the light will grow once more.

Self-Identity Ho'oponopono and Lomilomi: Self-Identity Ho'oponopono is a more modern process of ho'oponopono created by Morrnah Simeona, a well-respected kahuna from Honolulu, Hawaii. Her parents were Kimokeo and Lilia Simeona, both native Hawaiians. Her mother, Lilia, was one of the last recognized kahuna la'au kahea—a priest who heals with words. Morrnah was a practitioner of lomilomi and began to share her new form of ho'oponopono with the world in the 1970s. Through Morrnah's wisdom and insight, the process of ho'oponopono from ancient times was translated and developed into a more practical and effective tool for the world of today. Here is one prayer she offers for this process:

Divine Creator, Father, Mother, Son as One,

If I, my family, my relatives, and ancestors have offended you, your family, relatives, and ancestors, in thoughts, words, deeds, and actions, from the beginning of our creation to the present, we ask your forgiveness…

Let this cleanse, purify, release, cut all the negative memories, blocks, energies and vibrations and transmute these unwanted energies into pure light… And it is done.

The opening line first calls to the Divine, then calls into alignment a harmonized connection to the three aspects of our self, addressing them as Father, Mother, and Son as one. The prayer is then directed to anyone needing healing. It can be used for any relationship that needs clearing or balancing. It acknowledges the connection to the ancestors and appeals to them for their support in the forgiveness process.

The prayer is a call to direct the body (the child) to bring up any unhealthy energies needing to be transmuted into a higher vibration. The transmutation is done through a strong, clear prayer to spirit. Aunty Morrnah teaches us to invite the divine light to come down over us from above. This is the light of our own higher self, and the light of all of our ancestors. She asks the light to cleanse, transmute, and cut all ties to the negative memory. She closes with "It is done," to establish a clear and strong ending, affirming that it has indeed been transmuted.

Praying in this way was very effective for Aunty Morrnah's work, and there were many documented accounts of this prayer healing illnesses and other problems in people's lives. As more visitors arrived at the islands, she shared the system of ho'oponopono with them. Over time, the prayer was simplified and shortened into the form we commonly see today. The four lines used in this new forgiveness process are:

I'm Sorry. Please Forgive Me. Thank you. I Love You.

This seemingly simple prayer involves an interaction within our first circle of relationship—our personal soul cluster; the inner relationship between the 'unihipili (ku), the 'uhane (lono), and the 'aumakua (kane). When entering this process, the conscious mind gives a clear direction to the sub-conscious mind to bring to the surface anything that is still unforgiven in its memory bank. These unforgiven or unresolved memories can be seen as an unclean energy of a lower vibration. The 'unihipili uploads the energies of judgment, fear, resentment, guilt, anger, etc. 'Uhane then gives direction to the 'aumakua to send down grace to cleanse, purify, and transmute the lower energies into pure light.

For example: The words "I'm sorry" are directed toward the higher self from the lower self, apologizing for all its unclean baggage (such as judgment and resentment), and asking for forgiveness. The words "Please forgive me" are being used to ask the higher self to cleanse and release all unforgiven energies being held in the lower self. "Thank you" affirms your commitment and willingness to replace all unwanted energies with pure light. "I love you" is the closing that releases the prayer with full commitment to live in the spirit of aloha from that moment forward, in the freedom of everyone's absolute innocence.

As a giver of healing you can use this ho'oponopono prayer to help transmute the energy that your receiver has brought to you. To do this effectively, you take personal responsibility for what you perceive in the receiver as unclean or unresolved. It is a reflection of something that is also inside of you, and so you must address that part of you, and you transmute the memories in your own ku or 'unihipili.

In the acceptance of this shared process, the result is kala, a powerful release of energy blockages within both you and the receiver, making space for pure creative energy to flow in, and be used however you desire.

When you discover a hard or painful place on the body of your receiver, sometimes this is accompanied by unpleasant emotions. This means you have located a place where past trauma or crystalized judgments have been stored. As you come to these places pause, breathe, ground yourself, and silently acknowledge the presence of 'aumakua—a divinity within both you and the receiver.

Ask for cooperation from the 'unihipili (the body) to release the attachment to anything unforgiven, and transmute the energy into light. In these places of stored trauma, both giver and the receiver can speak the prayer, using a Ha breath, into that part of their body, giving the body permission to finally let go of it!

The ancestors can speak through you to the receiver and you will be guided via careful listening as to what style of lomi or quality of presence will create kala. Then you can proceed, asking the receiver to breathe their light and their love into this area with you. Sometimes it is helpful for the receiver to say aloud, "Whatever this is, I choose to forgive it. I let it go!"

It is not always necessary to know what it is that you are forgiving. The vibration of forgiveness is the ingredient in the lomi session that creates a crack in the crystallized memories where light can pour in and open things up for healing to be realized.

▽△▽△▽△▽△▽△▽△▽△▽△▽△▽△▽

EXERCISE: Clear Yourself with Self-Identity Ho'oponopono

Preparation: This exercise can be done seated comfortably, in a quiet place. It is a process of deep reflection and connecting to the divine, so you will need to be able to concentrate and be undisturbed. It may also help to think about the issues in your life that you would like to work with before starting and write down some specific things needing your forgiveness in a journal. This will help you to focus on one or two main issues in the exercise. You can also journal after the exercise and write down any shifts in perception that occur.

To begin: Open a clear connection to your higher self by breathing in the awareness of your own divinity, inhaling from above you into your belly, and exhaling with a Ha breath. Look inside your heart and feel around for any areas of your life or any relationships that may be harboring any hurt, such as feelings of judgment or resentment.

Bring your attention upward and ask your higher self to join with you and assist you to transform these feelings into pure divine light. Ask your higher self to help you see all situations in your life from a higher perspective. Now, direct your attention into your body, and give your body a clear directive to upload and release all energies of anger, fear, resentment, or guilt that needs clearing at this time, offering them up to your higher self. Allow whatever memories or sensations you are feeling to be fully felt and acknowledge them as they arise for clearing.

If it helps, you can place your hands on your body anywhere that you feel called to place them, so that you can communicate with your body more clearly. Take a deep breath, and say, "I'm sorry. Please forgive me." Allow any dense or unclean energy to come up to the surface.

Take another deep breath and then direct your attention upward, and draw in the light of your higher self to transmute the negative or unclean energy. Take as many breaths as needed to transmute the energy into pure divine light. Then say, "Thank you, I love you."

The process is like peeling back the layers of an onion. Once you start, you begin to unravel many layers of judgment and trauma stored within you. It is important to continue the process of ho'oponopono until you *feel* clear of these unclean energies in your feeling body, and to use it often, whenever needed, as hurtful things arise in your everyday life. In more difficult situations, you can call on the Holy Spirit, any of the ascended masters, angels, or God to intervene.

When situations in life trigger you, you can say the four lines quickly and flip your distorted, unclean perception into one of detached nonjudgment, innocent perception, and flow into compassionate disengagement.

The world around you will transform as you practice this. It will begin to respond to this new higher vibration you are transmitting in new and miraculous ways.

5

Pana—The Hidden Language of Life

Attentiveness and motion are the guardian
angels of the evolving consciousness.
—Kahu Abraham

To perform a lomilomi is to recognize and merge with the ancient rhythms of spirit in motion. When the kahuna speaks of ancient rhythms of spirit in motion, they are referring to *pana*. Pana literally means heartbeat, or a throbbing, pulsating rhythm. Pana is the hidden language of life, speaking through nature. Kahuna are taught to pay attention to everything around them, and to be attentive to the subtle changes in their surroundings. They listen to the birds, and analyze the tone of their songs. They watch their flight patterns, and determine their meaning. When out on the water, they feel the wind and watch the waves, reading the direction, the strength, the speed, merging in conscious ways with these natural rhythms. In this way, they learn to understand what all of nature is here to reveal. This acute awareness of energy in motion keeps them safe from storms or big changes in the environment and helps them find food and shelter when needed.

The ancient rhythms of spirit in motion flow through energetic patterns that unite all life forms—from the rhythm and motion of the precession of the stars and planets in our galaxy, to the movement of the tiniest bugs in the grass beneath us. These rhythms can be found in our bodies, in our breath, and in our heart beat. They can be seen in every aspect of nature, through careful observation. You can see them in the flight of a large flock of birds, a big school of fish swimming together as one, in the waves of the ocean and in the blowing wind across golden fields of grass. These primal rhythms connect us to a sense of complete unity and oneness with all of life, unfolding in every moment of our existence. These natural rhythms seen in nature have been tracked by ancient cultures from every corner of the globe, since before recorded time, and applied to healing the body, as a natural approach to medicine. The Hawaiian culture was one of the cultures that applied the ancient rhythms using bodywork techniques. In this chapter we will look at some primary sacred symbols, icons, and movements, and how they apply to bodywork.

The Wave

Life energy can be seen and measured in waves. In Hawaii it is easy to see these patterns as the tides rise and fall, and the different moods of the ocean speak so loudly. Ancient Hawaiians were great navigators—they invented surfing—and in so doing learned many things about the rhythm of life through the rhythm of the waves.

The ocean was also the primary source of food so their life was ocean-centric. In the training of Sherman Dudoit, his lomi kumu had him sit by the ocean for hours every day, squeezing sand between his hands while communing with the waves.

Uncle Harry was taught to observe the patterns of the waves, to count them, and witness the various patterns in the sets. He was taught much about life and healing through kayaking the rivers of Kauai. When you learn how to harmonize with the waves of the ocean, you can also apply that to riding the waves of life. There are many waves to look for in life, such as waves of emotion, waves of sensation, waves of activity, and waves of rest. All come to play in a lomi as you become the healing waves of pure aloha, washing up onto the shores of someone else's body.

All forms of life interact in waves of sound and light. As it blows across the surface of the ocean, wind co-creates waves with the moon, sun, and Earth's gravitational pull. As we inhale, our breathing creates waves of fresh energy coming in while toxins exit on the exhale. Even a thought creates energetic waves in this dimension. The process of creating life, as well as the process of death, and everything in between, involves interacting frequencies of energetic waves. When you apply the motion of the wave in your strokes during a massage, the body naturally responds by relaxing the tension it's holding.

The body surrenders to certain types of healing waves because it is the language of motion that it naturally attunes and relates to, much like a baby being comforted by a rocking motion or the gentle touch of a loving parent or grandparent. Love wants to blend with love. The lomi giver can create the perfect wave set or energetic vibration to match the waves being emitted by the receiver's organs. When these waves blend, the current changes and a transformation can then take place. You will even begin to see how waves occur as healing unfolds by being attentive to the subtle signals from your receiver's body. We call these waves of sensation. The waves of sensation follow a pattern of contraction followed by expansion, the natural waveform (pulse) through which all life recreates itself within our universe.

Rhythm

Lomilomi is a transmission, containing light and love, coming in the form of frequency vibration. A repeated frequency or pulse creates a rhythm. In training with Sherman Dudoit, we learned that when performing a Heartworks lomi, it's best to begin it with a steady rhythm. A repetitive stroke creates a vibrational pattern. When doing a shamanic healing session, you can tune into the rhythms of someone's body and adapt your technique to serve their need for releasing the tension from the body.

By focusing on the breathing pattern of the person receiving the treatment, you can coordinate your movements with the rhythm of their breath. You can tune into whatever speed or rhythm is most appropriate for the part of the body you are working on. Uncle Harry teaches that if we join the receiver at the bottom of the exhale, we can breathe along with them, deepening our connection to what they are experiencing as we stretch open and pull their body's extremities on their exhale.

The key to changing a pattern in the body is consistent repetition, as a stroke becomes more potent when repeated. In a massage, you repeat the stroke until the heat created from the friction softens the muscles. Sherman taught students to continue one repetitive stroke until they get lost in the rhythm of what he calls "love in motion," activating the transmission of divine light. The body relaxes into the rhythm because it is predictable and familiar. The mind relaxes into the rhythm because it is hypnotic and easy to follow. The mind surrenders to a deeper healing trance and the body relaxes, what we call moving through the layers. The rhythmic strokes and stretches move through the cell tissue and muscles much like water flowing through the rocks and channels of a mountain stream. The stress melts and the tension flows downstream toward the ocean.

Playing music during a healing session can influence the rhythm of your strokes too, affecting the receiver's ability to process what's happening. Be sensitive to the needs of the receiver. Adjust the music and the volume to suit their healing needs. If the music is too loud, you might become distracted or unable to hear or sense the receiver's breathing rhythm, missing the script all together. The right music at the right volume adds much to the healing trance experience.

The Spiral

The most common pattern in nature is the spiral; from the largest forms of creation, spiral galaxies, to helical patterns in human DNA. It is expressed in the Fibonacci sequence and comprises the golden ratio—everything in nature loves to move and grow and develop in a spiral formation. You can apply this to our own growth process to unlock nature's power in your life. As you grow, you spiral upward, each cycle building on the next, lifting you into a more mature version of yourself.

A growth cycle is like a spiral in which we move through contraction, expansion, and change. Throughout the cycles of our lives, we are required to revisit parts of ourselves that may need more healing. We encounter situations that trigger a feeling from childhood. The person who hurt you when you were young shows up with a different face but in a similar circumstance. It is at these intersections of growth and transformation that we can spiral. If we deal with it in a healthy way, we will spiral upward, while revisiting the old traumas from a more aware, enlightened perspective. As we heal the memory, it no longer holds the same energetic charge in our bodies. When we avoid the challenge, we do not heal, issues are not addressed, and we continue in the same old dysfunctional pattern as before. If we project our issue outward, we will tend to blame it on others. Or we may deal with the issue by trying to numb our feelings or escape from the pain in destructive and dysfunctional ways. When we do not face or release the root of an issue, we will spiral downward, causing more suffering, drama, or illness.

Knowing that all life evolves in spirals, you'll find that using spiraling movements can unwind and free up energy in the body. Our energy also flows through our chakras in a spiral motion. Because of this natural movement of all energy, stress and tension can be released from the body in a spiral pattern during a healing. This is also true within rotating the joints and the limbs. Much energy can be freed up and unblocked using this potent spiral motion throughout the healing. Sound can also enhance the movement of energy through the body's various energetic portals. Appropriately executed tones, singing, or various breathing patterns can also create a spiraling motion, assisting with removing blocked energy.

The Figure Eight

Another formation that opens and unlocks the universal flow of energy is the figure eight. In lomilomi, there are many strokes where the practitioner alternates with one hand and then the other hand; one clockwise and one counter clockwise. This alternating pattern is applied in a steady rhythm that balances the left and right sides of the brain, and unifies the masculine and feminine aspects of self. When applied over the heart area on the back of the body, this pattern can assist in balancing the body's energetic matrixes, while a deeper love is being infused into the cell memory. Later on, we will introduce the strokes that clean the rear heart chakra using alternating repetitive figure-eight strokes with the forearms and soft hands.

When repeated, the figure eight activates an energetic formation called the torus, a shape that is repeated everywhere throughout the universe. The torus is a three-dimensional geometric surface comprised of a closed curve that rotates around an axis but does not intersect it (think of the shape of a donut). Earth's torus is generated by the interaction of the magnetic fields of the north and south poles.

The torus is a very powerful figure that has been used to observe and harness free energy in motion by some brilliant scientists and inventors. Knowing that our energy and the energy of our planet naturally orbit in this formation helps us as healers to work with this same flow of energy in the body. The torus pattern can even be observed in our bodies around the electromagnetic field that pulsates outward from our hearts. Knowing this, we can use this pattern as a kind of *free energy generator* during a lomilomi massage.

The Cross—Horizontal and Vertical Connection

In addition to circles, spirals, and figure eights, in many lomi strokes we use corners or right angles as well as triangles and intersections, or crosses. Within these structures we discover that our strokes gain stability and focus. The places where lines of energy intersect on the body create points of focus for release, realignment, and integration.

The cross is one of the oldest and most common symbols in history. It has been used to show the four directions, four seasons, and four races of humankind, as well as the horizontal and vertical relationship of Earth's axis and the equator. The cross is also a symbol of the intersection between spirit and matter, or heaven and Earth. The horizontal represents the dimension of physical matter. Matter is dense and bound by gravity, space, and time. The vertical axis is the dimension of spirit. It is timeless and connected through all things; spirit has no density, gravity, time, or space.

The teachings of Kahuna Daddy Bray had to do with finding the balance between the spiritual and the material worlds. If we get too caught up in the mundane tasks of our everyday life, the horizontal, we feel trapped and life lacks any deep meaning. Likewise, if we spend too much of our time and energy with our head up in the clouds daydreaming or meditating on spiritual concepts, we may have a hard time focusing on the tasks of daily life and never achieve or fulfill our purpose in coming to Earth. Strive for living life in the center of the cross, where all things come together unifying the whole of creation, the zeropoint; this is the reason people meditate. Awareness is brought to this place at the center of the cross and requires stillness because we must focus our awareness on the only moment that actually exists. Spending a few minutes each day doing some form of meditation that brings you into the center of the cross will harmonize these opposite planes of existence and open you up to receive balanced guidance for bringing more spirit into matter and more heaven to earth.

Your role as the lomi giver is to anchor a vertical connection within the horizontal (physical) realm—connecting what is above with what is here below, receiving and channeling the Great Spirit's infinite energy into their healing. Most people are focused only on the horizontal earth plane, and this is their only problem. Your anchored connection to a spiritual realm will assist them greatly in reaching and experiencing a higher dimension within them. This draws them into an upward spiral—toward their light.

We spoke of living in the center of the cross, in balance between the material and the spiritual realms of life. The cross can be seen on the back of the body, with the spine as the vertical connection (our spiritual existence) and the shoulders as the horizontal connection (our earthly responsibilities). The center of the cross is over the heart, the *rear heart chakra*. To be focused on this center, where horizontal meets vertical, is to live in and from the heart, totally present. There are lomilomi strokes that join the horizontal plane of the shoulders with the vertical plane of the spine, harmonizing and balancing these connecting avenues of energy. The lomi strokes that open the shoulders soothe and release the stress we carry from our horizontal responsibilities, and the strokes that go up and down the spine promote the energy to flow more freely, connecting us to our higher function of being light in a body.

EXERCISE: Activating the Vertical and Horizontal Connection

Preparation: This exercise is to build energy and feel yourself in the center axis point in the cross, a bridge between heaven and earth. It can be done at any time to raise your energy, and is used to begin a prayer or ceremony or a healing activity such as bodywork. It can also just be used as a centering meditation, similar to qi gong. It will be most effective if your bare feet are planted firmly on the ground with your heels rooted into the earth's core along with your tailbone. Open the space between your legs by standing in what Serge King calls a *ku mana* power stance: Stand with your feet facing forward and parallel, shoulder-width apart, tailbone slightly tucked to flatten the lower back.

To begin: Place your awareness at the top of your head, feeling a connecting cord that reaches up, upward through dimensions all the way up into the heavens and the very center of our galaxy. Breathe in the energy from above down into your belly. Inhale with your attention above, and exhale with your attention at your navel. Then, notice your feet as they stand upon the ground.

Piko-piko (Center to Center) Breathing

Piko means "center." Feel a connecting cord going down into the very center of the earth you are standing upon. Feel the gravity of the earth, breathe, and pull the energy up from the earth, through the bottom of your feet into your belly—*piko*.

Now begin piko-piko breathing: alternate breathing in from above, and breathing in from below, feeling a channel of energy opening above and below you being directed into your physical body. Each breath, exhale at your navel to create a concentrated ball of pure love energy in your body, available to be used for healing.

You can piko-piko breathe from any point to any other point, energizing two centers to create a desired result. Your heart is the bridge and your hands become the extension of your heart—a vehicle for the energy of spirit to flow down from the vertical plane, descending into the horizontal plane. You can breathe in from above or below and then breathe out through your hands, allowing the mana to flow into a person, a space, an animal, or a tree. You can breathe to and from a star. Or you can place your hands on your own body and allow the mana to flow into a specific part of you, gathering mana, opening, expanding, and glowing in aloha light, and then exhaling it into the part of the body you are touching.

6

My Body, Your
Body, Our Body

The human body is a miraculous vehicle made of electric cosmic energy. It carries us and our immortal light until it is time for the light to depart, returning our soul to its dimension of origin. The physical body is a complex organic machine of fire, water, flesh, and bones. It is the infusion of our soul's light that creates companionship between spirit and flesh. Your body's many parts, operating as a family, will mirror your thoughts, beliefs, and the world around you. Keeping your self-healing vehicle-for-light functional requires a bit of self-care. Let's explore this a little further.

"My body" refers to the view of the external perspective of our flesh-and-bone machine. Getting to know the human body begins with getting to know the various parts of the body and the functions and needs that each one has in the family. "Your body" refers to your personal relationship with the physical vehicle. Consciousness is the bridge between your physical, mental, and spiritual space of existence. When you develop a strong connection to your body through loving self-care and mindfulness, you become open to more clear inspirations and higher vibrational frequencies from your higher self. You can also access the messages coming from the bodies of the people around you and help them hear their body's voice. "Our body" refers to how we are all connected to and affected by the one body of humanity living on one planet, in one galaxy, in one universe. Humankind can be viewed as having one giant human oversoul that's growing and maturing within many bodies, each one affected by everything that happens on earth. This is how your body can be used to access all times, all places, and all people. We can learn to influence all things through frequency, through the "spirit channel" in meditation or guided shamanic journeys. In these trance states, we connect deeply within cosmic consciousness beyond the boundaries of the body.

My Body: Developing a Conscious Mind-Body Relationship

There is a view of the body in which all of its individual parts are subject to what's going on within the whole three-fold being. This view holds that our body is a microcosm of the earth as well as the universe. This idea has created the demand for holistic health education, which acknowledges and promotes these simple ideas:

1. The body works as a family, with many parts sharing responsibility for the well-being of the whole.

2. What you feed your body—on every level—will affect all its parts. "Feeding" in this sense refers not only to food but also vibrations, beliefs, attitudes, projections, guilt, shame, resentments, and judgments.

3. Your habitual thoughts and states of mind will directly affect your body's health and performance from moment to moment. Change your thoughts and beliefs, and your body's performance will change.

4. The body has a voice. It is possible to communicate with your body to discover what it needs to be healthy, vibrant, and productive. If you do not listen to your body and keep pushing it in a direction it doesn't want to go, it can bring you down and make you feel ill or out of balance. When it's not receiving enough quality attention, it may create pain to get the attention it needs from you to make a change.

5. Our immortal spirit is infinitely powerful and can heal any illness, yet the body's healing is subject to our will to heal our emotional environment. Even if you are a skilled surgeon or gifted shaman, it's wise to acknowledge the fact that it is the frequency of pure unconditional love that recreates well-being in its own time.

The Body as 'Ohana

Kahu Abraham spoke about the body's nature as 'ohana as the most basic of all Hawaiian principles; he would say, "*everything in existence is family.*" He would talk about how all universes, planets, stars, animals, plants, and humans are all family. If you look at the physical body more consciously from the inside, you see that it too operates in much the same way a family does. Every member of the family has a role to play that benefits the whole body. Your body's systems—muscular, digestive, respiratory, skeletal, immune, endocrine, urinary, and reproductive—are all family systems that interact with each other and support the wellness of your whole body.

When all the family members are getting along, getting what they need—primarily love, acknowledgement, and nutrition—you may experience physical health. When you are not physically well, chances are one or more family members may require special attention to realign, recharge, or regenerate.

Kahu would say that every member of the family has a voice and deserves expression; that it is up to us to determine which family member is expressing itself to bring our attention to discover what it needs to perpetuate a harmonious well-being of the whole.

In our healing practice, we have found that for almost everyone, the body-mind connection has been somewhat overlooked, and that there is no real conscious relationship between the two. It's safe to say that most people are generally unaware of what their body is up to. Until they experience some form of pain that captures their attention, they just don't understand what a conscious relationship—offering consistent praise and self-maintenance—will offer them.

The Body as a Domain

Kahu would say that your body is a kingdom or queendom; the key word here being "your." Abraham often used the metaphor of a body as a domain, with your mind as the ruler of the domain. Within your body, all the subjects of your realm reside. Here's where the personal relationship begins. Once ownership of the domain has been established, the responsibilities of stewardship—an intimate, loving relationship and the protocols for proper care—can begin. Kahu's metaphor works very well to illustrate how all the family members have a primal codependent relationship based upon acknowledgment, trust, and mutual respect. The following excerpt from Abraham's lecture demonstrates this:

> Acknowledgement begins with yourself. As an example, imagine yourself as a domain, a realm, of which you are the ruler and every cell within your body are your subjects. All the different parts of your body are your subjects. For years, your subjects have toiled day and night to perpetuate this domain, to perpetuate this realm, this kingdom or this queendom, this nation of You. If you spent a little time talking to your body, touching your body, addressing your body as though it were a being, it will definitely respond to you. If you do

not, then you as the ruler of the domain of self will have a conflict on your hands. Let's say, one day you have this great idea of going on a great crusade towards higher consciousness, towards greater spirituality, and you get out to the balcony and all the subjects of your realm are there. Do you think as a personal human being, you would follow anyone who does not acknowledge you? As a human being, would you follow this ruler or anyone who cannot give you a compliment, all your life?

When you develop a relationship with your body that's based on consistent care and loving attention, kahuna wisdom teaches that the body will become an eager servant to the mind. The body is wise, intuitive, and powerful; when it is treated with consideration and kindness, it will happily give you whatever is needed for any task or project.

Take a moment now to ask yourself:

+ As the King or Queen of my domain, what kind of ruler am I?

+ Do I criticize and punish, or do I lovingly support, guide, and nurture with respect, as a good ruler would?

+ What kind of relationship do I as a King or Queen have with the subjects of my realm? Do I listen to their needs, or do I just give orders?

+ Do I take the subjects of my realm for granted until I'm in pain?

✦ Have I ever communicated with my organs to find
out what is required for optimizing or improving
functionality?

EXERCISE: Self-Care—A One-Week Exploration

The subjects of your realm need to feel acknowledged
and appreciated in order to give you more than they
are giving you already. Just try this practice for one
week and see what happens. See what happens when
you approach it with a loving sincerity, a cooperative
dialogue, and easy aloha.

Preparation: This exercise takes one week, so you
can decide when you would like to do this, and mark it
on your calendar. You will need a journal to write about
each day, recording your progress in the following areas:
Exercise, Water, Food, Blessings. In these areas, be sure
to write what you actually did that day, how you felt
about it emotionally, and the way your body responded
to your attention. Also, write down what you think your
body might be saying to you, and see if you can tune
into what your body is telling you it needs.

To begin: For seven days, you will be consciously
working in the body in a new way. Strive to try a new way
of doing things and to let your body guide you in your
activities. Improve or expand your exercise program sub-
stantially. When you move your body, be aware. Rather

than forcing your body to move, ask your body how it wants to move. Put on some music and try moving your body around freely, just letting it guide you. Each day, choose a form of exercise that your body is calling for, and do it with joy!

Improve the quality of food you eat and water you drink. Ask your body if that is what it wants before consuming anything, and eat mindfully. Eat slowly and chew your food twice as long as you would normally. For one week between meals, drink more water than you would normally drink at other times.

Now add a personal daily dialog, a constant flow of blessings. Say "I love you" to your body, acknowledging any areas needing care and appreciation. Do this while relaxing in bed every morning and evening.

For one week, write down what happens each day: how your body feels, makes requests, and responds. Has anything shifted or come to the surface? Is your body telling you anything? Remember to listen to your body and also respond to it with gentleness. You are developing a bridge between your conscious and subconscious minds.

Training Your Body

Once you develop a strong mind-body connection, you can train your body to do great things. Let's use an Olympic athlete as the example. Athletes train for several years, holding their body in the highest regard and esteem. They are acutely aware that in order to get their body to do everything they want it to do, they have to take the very best care of it in every possible way. It is the quality of this primary relationship with their mind, body, and spirit that will determine their physical performance in the Olympic games.

Athletes also use positive visualizations and declarations as part of programming their body to do things that the average human body cannot do! They repeatedly run perfect-patterns of performance in their minds, which trains their inner-body to perform their chosen routine perfectly. Seventy percent of an Olympic athlete's training takes place in their mind visualizing the perfect performance over and over again. They are programming their body for the perfect performance, having learned that the body is a pattern-oriented machine that works on the basis of running patterns successfully and receiving rewards. Healing works in the same way.

Holistic health is the science of consciously attending to, loving, and appreciating all parts of you as one family. Each member of the family has specific needs and an intrinsic role to play in the success of your overall health and performance. Consider practicing a positive visual programming next time you're about to begin a difficult task, such as meeting with someone you have a conflict with, doing something physically challenging, or attending an important meeting, so you can clear the way beforehand for a beneficial outcome for all involved. Before you begin the challenging task, just sit, close your eyes, and see yourself doing the task. See it being done with ease and grace. Call in your higher self to do the task for you. Do not begin the task until you have filled your body with the feelings of ease and grace. Using these mind skills, you can clean and clear the pathway before going into any important process with visual, prayerful aspirations and gratitude.

▽△▽△▽△▽△▽△▽△▽△▽△▽△▽△▽△▽△

EXERCISE: Blessing Your Body—A Self-Healing Meditation

Preparation: The very best relationship to have with your body for optimum health is cultivated through consistent acknowledgment and blessings. Move or stretch on the floor for several minutes to open up your body before beginning. This exercise is best done sitting or lying comfortably with loose clothing, so that you can really get into healing your body. You can move or touch your body in any way you feel is most healing as you do the exercise.

To begin: Relax and close your eyes, taking in three deep Ha breaths. On the first breath as you inhale, collect the energy of appreciation and respect within you. On the exhale, offer your appreciation and respect to your physical body. On your second inhale, breathe in deep appreciation and respect. Then as you exhale, offer appreciation and respect to your intellect (your mind). On your third breath, inhale deeply the energy of loving appreciation and respect. On a slow exhale, offer love, appreciation, and respect to your higher self and your ancestors. Repeat this whole process three times.

Next we add touching, feeling, and blessing your body to this process, beginning with your feet, at the tips of your toes. Touch and extend your love into the cells of your feet using your breath. Breathe deeply as you tune into every part of your toes, feet, and ankles. Allow enough time and space to listen to what your feet have to say to you. Breathe your love into each one of the cells of your feet. Continue this pattern of breathing your love into the body's cells, offering your appreciation by talking to the cells, and listening to what the cells have to say to you, while touching and massaging your feet, breathing love into them.

Do this for your whole body, slowly working your way up into your ankles, calves, and knees, up into your thighs and hips. Bless each hip one at a time. The right hip is a connecting point to the masculine ancestors. When you come here, take a moment to offer blessings to your father and grandfathers here. The left hip is a connecting point to the feminine ancestors. Take a moment to offer blessings to your mother and grandmothers here. Breathe your love into every cell of your body, slowly working your way up into your stomach. Touch and massage your stomach, moving through every part of your colon with appreciation and respect.

Bless every muscle, organ, and bone in your upper torso. Be sure to include the stomach, intestines, liver, heart, lungs, kidneys, ribs, spine, arms, hands, and fingers.

Bless each shoulder one at a time. Acknowledge the connection to the divine masculine as you touch your right shoulder, the altar of the grandfathers. This shoulder is a connecting point to your masculine ancestors. Then acknowledge the connection to the divine feminine as you touch your left shoulder, the altar of the grandmothers. When you are ready, you can move up to your neck.

Continue this pattern of breathing divine love into all your cells, offering your appreciation and gratitude by talking to them, telling them that you love them. Listen to what they have to say while touching and massaging your whole body, one family member at a time. Be sure to touch every part of your face and skull, and bless your brain, ears, teeth, jaw, skull, and hair.

When you have thoroughly blessed every part of your body, take three deep Ha breaths again: one breath for your body, one for your mind, and one for your spirit. Take a moment while lying flat on your back on the floor to feel the amazing sensations of aliveness running through your whole body. Allow a little time for a sacred reunion of the family. Breathe and expand into this healing blessing for your whole body and all the subjects of your realm.

When this exercise is performed effectively, you will feel a glow or a tingling warmth from within and around your body. Your body will always respond to your loving attention. When you feel fulfilled and at peace in this practice, arise slowly. Take this glow with you into your day ... or your dreamtime.

Your Body: Working to Reframe, Re-parent, and Take Responsibility

Become more aware of the family of relationships within yourself and how your communication skills affect your overall health and performance. Then you will be able to assist others to become aware not only of the subtle messages they are receiving from their own bodies, which can be obvious if they are in any kind of pain, but also of the messages they are feeding to their body on a regular basis via their thoughts, feelings, and unconscious habits and behaviors. For example, someone may come complaining of a bad shoulder, weak knee, or painful wrist. They may say, "This is my bad shoulder." You can ask them politely to please rephrase what they have just said to give the cells within their shoulder—the subjects of their realm—a more conscious, positive, vibrational feeling. *For example:* "This is my good shoulder that I love so much. It's having a challenge right now but it's getting better, and I am willing to forgive whatever is causing the pain."

A big part of helping others to heal involves helping people learn to "re-parent" themselves. We need to empower people to develop healthy and loving relationships with their own bodies. Sometimes, many of us tend to behave as if we are led by our body's moods—our happiness becomes subject to how it's doing or feeling. Other times, we will behave as an overbearing parent in relationship to our body. How many times have you given your body criticism or forced it to do something it didn't want to do or was not properly prepared for? As parents in our family dynamic, we tend to want our children to be a certain way for *our own* comfort and benefit. Most of us who have had children know it is very difficult to be a loving parent when dealing with a child who is radically misbehaving. We just want them to obey, and it's hard not to get angry when they don't. Likewise, we sometimes treat our bodies the way we might treat our kids. We give orders and expect them to be followed. Why? Because our mind thinks it is in control regarding our domain. We want the body to carry out whatever we want it to do even though it may not be ready, willing, or able to do so.

It is better to be a fair, loving, cooperative parent who develops an intimate relationship with the body—one of mutual respect. Learn to ask your body nicely to do something and then listen carefully for its fears, resistance, and concerns. Keep in mind the royalty analogy: when your subjects feel heard, they bring more cooperation to the task at hand, and any fear or resistance pattern will subside. This quality of attention will build trust among all the family members; spiritual, physical, and emotional. Your subconscious mind holds much power when it comes to the process of manifesting your desires.

As a healer, you may become so skilled at listening and communicating with your own body that it naturally develops your ability to listen and communicate with the body of another. This practice awakens your empathic nature, and you will begin to feel what the other is feeling. With plenty of attentive practice, their body will speak loud and clear to you after a while, and it will tell you exactly what it needs for an optimal release. You can merge so deeply with another in a healing that their body will hear and feel everything you are thinking and transmitting through your touch as well. Your thoughts, vibrations, and healing intentions will be felt in the body of the receiver, and they will respond by coming into alignment with a higher frequency of vibration, of which you are generating with love, respect, and humility from your own space of existence.

The Body Has a Voice

Losing a loved one or being hurt can often trigger a traumatic emotional response. Even if it's processed with the utmost care, the residue of trauma is stored in the body, often in the organs, the shoulders, and/or the lower back. The aka (energetic cords running between you and them) can become frayed, broken, or clogged and filled with darker emotions like grief, judgment, hatred, anger, and resentment. This unhealthy connection becomes a drain on your life force, which over time will bring pain because your energy has become toxic. Toxicity can create distortions, walls, or holes in your energy field. If you are spending more energy hating than you actually have available to spend, you may become energetically bankrupt in that particular relationship.

By acknowledging and forgiving yourself and the others involved, perhaps within a ho'oponopono or a truth dialog, you clear the stuck, crystalized yuck (toxin) from the emotional body. After untangling the emotional and mental issues, these things can be relieved from the physical body, assisted by a breathing session or bodywork treatment.

There are many ways the body communicates. The body begins by telling us things quietly, through sensations, emotions, and intuitive feelings, fears, and ideas. Over time, if we ignore the quiet messages of the body, it will begin to try other ways to get our attention, by attracting some pain or even illness. Eventually, the body acts like a stubborn child, throwing a fit, and unwilling to let go of something until its needs have been met. Once again, family dynamics play into every aspect of the healing process. It is up to you to help others to uncover what the body, mind, and spirit are communicating, or not communicating.

Quite often when the body is acknowledged in a way that it understands or can feel heard and accepted, it will begin to let go of pain immediately. The Great Spirit wants you to have what you truly desire, and your body will guide you toward this pursuit if you surrender to the process. In this way, pain can be our greatest teacher, revealing to us what needs to be allowed for us to have what we want. It will give us clues when we've closed our heart and encourage us to open it again with unconditional loving attention. Use the pain as a way to get to the root of the emotional issue taking place under the surface.

For example, the body may be holding a pattern from the hurt inner child such as, "I am scared. I don't feel safe" or "It feels like my dad (or mom, or other prominent parental figure) does not love me." These messages are learned patterns from childhood and are deeply ingrained. It is very healing to address the inner child and uncover what it's trying to reveal and release. Using prayer and/or meditation can help you look deeper into the psyche and communicate with that part of the person who is hurting. You can work with your clients and teach them how to speak directly to their own inner child, a great skill to practice. Listen carefully and respond as a responsible parent to what the "inner child" needs with unconditional love and acceptance.

Our Body—Beyond the Flesh

The universe can be accessed and influenced by communication through the body. The same conscious substance that makes up the stars also makes up our body. The entire universe can be accessed by looking within, because within each one of us, exists a connecting chord to the center of the universe. Your body is made of the same substance as everything on Earth. Carbon-based units filled with electrical currents (spirit) animate and support life. These electrical currents are sourced by an infinite supply of energy that is highly intelligent and highly creative. The source of all life operates through all things to create and hold in place an immaculate reality for us all to thrive in while exploring the mysteries of our bodies.

Meditation or shamanic journey takes us into our body through our breath. We shut out all outer stimulation and move inward. When we are deep in meditation or in a visionary trance, the boundary of our body disappears and it is as if a portal opens inside us, and we begin to move beyond our body. Our consciousness enters a higher dimension, and we find that we are in a limitless expansive space. From this open state of awareness, our spirit can travel to other times or other places. We can connect with other people on the level of spirit. This is how remote healing takes place. When we heal something on the inner plane, it can affect our whole family, because their bodies are connected to ours. In this heightened state of consciousness, we can also communicate with higher beings, the spirit world, and feel a stronger connection to God, communing with divinity. Shamans use these trance states to influence the healing of the earth, other people, or to gain a greater understanding of the workings of spirit. This is often called the dreamtime.

The Earth Is Our Body

Just as the environment around us affects our body, what we see in the world around us is also a reflection of our inner reality. When we see toxic issues in the environment such as war, nuclear meltdowns, oil spills, hurricanes, floods, or forest fires, we look within for answers to these problems. Although these environmental issues *seem* outside of us and beyond our control, we can take responsibility for our own inner environment—cleaning up the toxic mess we created within our own lives—in our body or in our mind. Next time you see something disturbing on the news, try asking yourself, "How does what I see in the world exist within me?" If you see war, look at your relationships to see where you can create more peace. Then begin cleaning your perception with self-identifying ho'oponopono. If you see environmental issues, look into your physical health and ask what you can do to create more harmony or detoxify your body and your home. Everything in the outer world changes as you change yourself.

The outside world is a mirror, reflecting what is going on inside of us, because we are truly one. We are the earth, we are made up of her essence and she sustains our life with her love. When we take care of our own bodies, the world around us transforms, reflecting the wholeness we have fostered within ourselves.

As a bodyworker, you will train yourself to listen more deeply to your own body as well as the bodies of others to hear what they are ready to reveal to you, in order for you to know just what depth of pressure or what to say to crack open the armor around their heart, or what quality of acknowledgment is required to significantly reduce or release the emotional and/or physical pain that they are holding onto. When working deeply on someone's body in a lomilomi massage, moving very slowly through a stroke with absolute attentiveness, you can actually feel what the other is feeling. Their body will tell you how to execute each stroke, at what speed, and at what depth of pressure. Your body and their body has become "our" body in that very moment, as an immortal healing presence flows into and through both the giver and the receiver. This is how you as a lomi giver or health practitioner are healed in the practicing of this transformational work.

When your client's vibration raises from low to high and their awareness heightens, it will affect all areas of their life as they return home, and those dear to them will feel the healing rippling into them as well. In other words, everyone in your client's life will be affected on some level by what just happened to them in your healing temple. The animals, plants, waters, and rocks pick up on this higher vibration. The earth is transformed as we love ourselves and each other. Your sincere efforts of healing yourself and others ripples waves of freedom and peace far and wide, extending throughout infinity to everyone and all universes in all dimensions.

7

The Body and Lomilomi

To combine the Spiritual and the Material is the most
important teaching the kahuna can give the world.
—Kahuna David Bray

In a full lomilomi massage (with oil), the practitioner typically
works the whole body, from back to front. Much attention is
paid to the body as a whole being, and many of the strokes
serve to integrate all parts of it. This chapter is dedicated to
the body, working from the head down to the toes, offering a
variety of ways to view and work with the body. We hope some
of the ideas and information here will inspire you to go deeper
into the miraculous realm of the human body. Though rooted
in Hawaiian teachings, these ideas are eclectic, effective tools,
taken from our direct experience of learning, giving, and receiving lomi as shamanic bodywork.

Po'o (Head)

The head is related to the mind and your thoughts. It is said that all illness begins with a thought, and so all healing must also begin with a thought. It is imperative to relax the mind for healing to take place, so anything done to soothe the head or skull helps the mind to relax, sending this message to the entire nervous system.

A little scalp massage goes a long way to relax the taut mind of someone really stressed. Sometimes the script will require you to start a session with a firm, deep scalp massage in order for a hyperactive mind to relinquish control. Only then will it allow the body to relax, so they can enjoy the massage.

In the upper dimensions, the realm of light in Hawaiian is called *'Ao*, and the realm of darkness, *Po*. In traditional lomi, the head is called *Po'o*. *Po* is also the Hawaiian word for the realm of the "un-manifest" where all life originates. When un-manifest becomes manifest, it begins to reflect light, birthed from Po, concentrated into a physical form, bringing it into the realm of the manifest. When the kahuna speaks of working on the skull, he says to look for the light in the darkness. Inside the skull, it is very dark, and yet there is so much activity going on inside the brain; every thought is a spark of light in the darkness that has now come to life. In traditional lomi there are various techniques used on the head. Attention is paid to the plates of the skull, feeling for any swelling, bumps, or tight areas, gently massaging and manipulating the plates of the skull to open, clear, and release any traumas or blocked energy. Then the energy can flow freely through the top of the head, opening pathways to the light of the spirit. The occipital bone is a very significant area—a portal to the soul.

Helelena (Face)

The face is a reflection of our thoughts and beliefs about ourselves. It displays our moods and how we present ourselves to the world. It develops as we grow older. A traumatized child will hold tension patterns in their face. When we look at ourselves in the mirror, we often project unloving thoughts. Learn to look into your eyes in the mirror and see into your own soul. Accept and love all that you see. It is very powerful to do this as a daily practice. It can be a profound experience for anyone who has been projecting negative affirmations and harsh judgments onto themselves.

You can learn a lot about a person by looking at their face. Our thought patterns shape our face as we age. You may notice some people seem to have a permanent frown. Others have lines from years of joy and laughter. Some people have lines from years of physical or emotional pain. Others have a big difference between the left and right sides of their face, which speaks of an imbalance between their inner masculine and feminine. The face transforms and reveals many things during a healing session. It helps to watch the face of the client when possible while working on other parts of the body, as it will show you when they are releasing (sighing, laughing, or crying), when they are contracting (holding the breath, tightening facial muscles), and when they are expanding (smiling, relaxing, breathing deeply).

A good face massage can remove years of stress, leaving the client looking younger and healthier. With a shamanic approach to face massage, we can remove the masks the person has worn in the world, the façade of the false self, and uncover their more authentic nature. It is important when working the face to pay attention to the jaw. The jaw may need clearing, as it can hold a lot of tension. This area connects directly to speaking one's truth. It may be necessary for the client to give a voice to things they have needed to say, but felt unsafe to say, in order to release the tension. In this book we share ways of doing facial massage as a shamanic ritual. This process consciously engages the client and reprograms their brain as you clear their face.

'A'i (Neck)

Carrying the weight of our head is a big job! The head is a fairly large and heavy object, and the neck is responsible for balancing and supporting it all day long. Rotating the head, and stretching and massaging the neck are good methods of relief from the heaviness of daily stress. There are many specific moves that we teach to help release tension in the neck. The neck can be seen as a bridge between the mind and the body, so we need to keep this area free of blockages. The neck is the bridge between the brain—the command center—and the rest of the body.

The neck also encompasses the throat and the voice. If there is an issue in the neck it is important to look at what words are not being spoken. It may be that the client needs to express some heartfelt feelings, but they are holding back for fear of hurting another. Having the client speak these feelings into the sacred space you have created for them and perhaps make a sound that comes from their very soul can help unblock the neck and throat area, using their emotional body to express the release.

Po'ohiwi (Shoulders)

The shoulders are associated with the horizontal plane. This is where we carry our personal kuleana (responsibilities); work, family, and relationships. The shoulder blades often carry stress and tension which sometimes feels like rocks or like carrying "the weight of the world." In the realm of massage, we realize this is often the case for upper back tension. Shoulder problems are sometimes caused by repetitive strain from a type of job that hurts the body. The body is trying to tell the person to stop what they are doing, but the person keeps going, creating or aggravating an injury.

Problems in the shoulder can also be caused by memories held in the bones. Because there are so many nooks and crannies in the shoulder, there are many places where hurtful memories can lodge. Following are some deep joint rotations to pull the crystallized memories out of the shoulder joint, down the arms, and out through the hands. With a blanket of forgiveness, we can clear anything, so it's not all that important to know exactly what issue is trapped in the shoulder. To apply the blanket of forgiveness, have the person focus on the area of pain and say the words, "Whatever this is, I choose to forgive it now. Whatever is causing this pain, I set it free!" While holding the person's shoulder, you can rapidly mumble the words, "This shoulder is releasing, this shoulder is releasing" over and over while working the area that's holding onto the pain. By repeating the words with a loving conviction, the body begins to follow your soft yet firm commands.

Kuamo'o (Spine)

The spine represents our vertical connection to source. Kealohi calls this area "the highway of Christ energy." By this, he means this is the pathway of divine light, traveling up and down the body through intricate nerve systems, giving all of the body direction and information through electrical impulses. Our spine is our inner support system, so it reflects how we feel about ourselves and how we run our lives. You can learn a lot from someone's posture. Does the person hunch over, attempting to protect their heart? Do they lean forward, as if rushing through life or living in the future? Or do they lean back out of fear or suspicion?

Do they stick out their belly and crunch their lower lumbar, giving to the point of draining themselves, without keeping themselves balanced? Is their spine stiff, swollen and/or rigid, expressing fear, reflecting inflexibility, stubbornness, or unwillingness to forgive? Is the spine soft, curved, wobbly, or prone to going out of place, reflecting instability, restlessness, or neediness? If there is something out of place in the spine, it can disrupt or displace the energy of the entire body. Athletes know this only too well. By aligning the vertebrae of the spine, it is possible to relieve pain and increase your energy, mental clarity, relaxation, and flow. Each vertebra connects to a specific organ of the body, so as you open and clear the spine, the whole body receives healing.

Deep, slow lomi strokes moving up and down the spinal processes with your power pad and/or your elbow open the way for more light or electrical current to flow through the body, a method called spinal irrigation. People will look much younger after a good lomi session, because when the spinal column is deeply irrigated, the receiver's nervous system opens, clearing their whole body through the "highway" of the spine's electrical system with potent waves of aloha light. We use specific breathing patterns as we apply deep elbow strokes for clearing the body's electrical running system along the spine. The up and down, slow irrigation process nicely enlivens and awakens the ebb and flow of the kundalini energy from Earth to heaven through the whole body. The spine connects to the rib cage and all the muscles that support the back. The back can be seen as a protective shell for the vital organs. The ribs surrounding the heart can store crystallized memories that need releasing using bone washing. The strokes in lomilomi often spread outward from the spine, opening the space between the vertebrae, ribs, and surrounding muscles.

Opu (Belly)

The belly is a very important part of most Hawaiian healing as the belly area is said to be the center of personal power. Your ku is centered here and communicates its messages through your belly. This area is known as the seat of our emotions, or the basket of emotions. The wisdom of the ku is communicated through feelings that are felt in the belly. This is where our gut feelings and intuition are generated and expressed. In Hawaiian, gut knowledge is called *na'au*.

The part of our body that completes the processing of our food, separating the nutrients from the waste materials is seated here, the colon. All the food we eat is processed through our digestive system, and nutrients are distributed throughout the entire body. It is an amazing process that involves all the organs working together as a family. When there is an upset in one member of the family of our digestive system, it can throw the balance off in the whole body. When we take care of the colon, we take care of our entire being. Much of Hawaiian plant medicine is related to cleansing the colon. The processing of fear or unresolved resentments or guilt goes along with clearing toxins from the body. For any definitive healing to sustain, it is important to address the client's diet and nutrition. We need to pay attention to what we are eating when we are stressed—some foods we think will *ease* our stress can actually increase our stress exponentially.

We need to pay attention to what we are eating when we are stressed—some foods we think will ease our stress can actually increase it exponentially. This is often the case when the ileocecal valve is stuck open, recycling toxins back into the body, When overwhelmed by too much stress, the ileocecal valve becomes over sensitive to spices, acidic foods, alcohol, caffeine and grain rough-age. So, what is "healthy" to eat becomes relative to the condition of the colon. We actually teach adjustments for this condition.

Aka (Energetic Connections)

The navel area is sometimes said to be the center from which we send out aka, energy that connects us to everything we place our attention on. Information travels to our bodies through the aka. Through the aka we are able to feel the feelings of others, the connection to the higher self in those around us, and our ancestors. The belly is where we hold our "bowl of light" as explained in the last chapter. In it we can carry the stones of anger, guilt, shame, or blame, leaving less space for light. Our Hawaiian teachers reminded us that all you have to do is Huli' the bowl—turn it over! The rocks fall out, and your light can shine fully once again. There are some great massage moves for the belly that assist with this process. This type of stomach lomi is called Huli Ka Opu. Much attention is paid to the belly with a variety of moves that follow the flow of digestion, massaging the liver and stomach in a circular motion. The deep massage techniques cleanse the entire length of the colon, releasing emotional and physical blockages. Specific maneuvers adjust and align the intestinal valves and organs so that anything stuck or out of place returns to its proper position.

Iwi (Bones)

The bones carry our mana, the spiritual essence of our being because mana is stored in bone marrow. Likewise, Hawaiian people took great care in the preparing and wrapping of the bones of their deceased ancestors and chiefs. The spirit of the deceased person was thought to live on in their bones. The bones of important people were carefully hidden in far-off caves so no one could mess with the spirit of that person after leaving the body. In traditional lomi, it is taught that memories are stored in the skin of the bone, the fiber surrounding the bone, attaching to tendons, fascia, or muscle. Later, we will share the technique of bone washing, which releases crystallized memories from the surface of the bone, moving it out the extremities.

Papakole (Hips)

The hips are connected to the pelvis and the sacrum, serving as a base to our structure, and housing our reproductive organs. The issues associated with the hips or pelvis are usually related to sex; money; stability; and family relationships, such as one's grandparents, spouse, or one's children. Our root chakra also deals with your issues around safety, survival, and security. Some say that the ancestors communicate through the hips; the right side would be associated with masculine relations, left side would be feminine relations.

In Temple Style lomi we do deep joint rotations for the hips that open and unblock energy being stored in the hip joints, pelvis, and sacrum area. The sacrum area also holds many treasures. Some teachers call this area the "well of our being." I was taught that it stores the blueprint relating to our soul's purpose, as well as connections to our children (born and unborn). It is important to massage the entire sacrum area deeply, gently, tenderly. There are many ligaments and muscles that connect around the edges of the sacrum—a worthy navigation for comforting your receiver. Lomilomi often involves massaging the buttocks, and working the contours of the pelvis, releasing the tension in the psoas muscle.

Wawae (Feet and Legs)

The feet are a primary part of our root structure that symbolizes the way we carry ourselves, our direction (or lack of it), and how we get ourselves there. They relate directly to the way in which we connect to the earth's energy. Issues in the feet such as fallen arches will create a misalignment in the hip, spine, neck, and jaw. People with a short leg will also have this challenge. Pay attention to the feet whenever possible, and notice how the client is standing. This affects the alignment of the whole body. Is the entire foot firmly on the ground? How strong and flexible are the ankles? Are the feet turned too inward or outward? Notice now whether the person is leaning on the left (the feminine) or the right (the masculine). All these things are a reflection of how a person sees him or herself and navigates this world.

In a lomi session, we work the legs thoroughly. There are deep knee rotations from Kahu's teaching that open and release stuck energy. Uncle Harry explained that the calves were called the "second heart" because they pump so much blood and oxygen through the body. He taught us to work just the legs and feet, about forty minutes per leg, with the receiver lying on their back. This is known as *kala'e*, which means "clearing the rivers." In doing this we learned to clear from the hip, all the way down the leg, and out the feet and toes. When you spend a long time working on one part of the body, transformation takes place in the whole being.

The lomi strokes for the foot can relieve many ailments and assist the flow of unwanted energy to leave the body. Later in this book we share a blessing ritual that combines an interactive dialog and footbath, deeply clearing each foot as we clear the mental and emotional bodies. When massaging the feet, it is important to pay close attention to every muscle, bone, and tendon—as well as every toe. It is helpful to use a spiraling motion to rotate the ankles and toes deeply, very slowly. This relieves some of the pressure from carrying the weight of the whole body.

Manamana Lima (Hands and Arms)

The hands symbolize our connection to the heavens. They resemble the spreading branches of a tree. The hands are how we bring the gifts of our ancestors and spirit to the world around us, how we engage in our communities. Hands are often associated with giving and receiving. In many shamanic schools, the left hand (feminine,) is associated primarily with receiving, and the right hand (masculine) is associated primarily with giving. This idea can be useful in sacred ceremony and also in healing work, although in reality both hands are always giving and receiving.

Spreading open each hand to channel more light is very effective medicine. In a lomi session we open and massage the center of the palm of each hand deeply, thoroughly, and pull and clear each finger, releasing stress throughout the entire body. When the hands are blocked, there is nowhere for stagnant energy to get out. It is common for the traditional lomi kumu to begin a session with opening the hands and the feet of the receiver before working on the rest of the body.

Hands receive information in the form of energy. Our computer-centric culture produces stressed forearms and hands, as do factory, construction, and service industry jobs. So we massage and clear the entire length of the arm, from the shoulder, down the arms to the hands and out the fingertips.

Be attentive. If the client's hands have energy but are feeling tight and stressed, the person is likely overworked, giving too much away and not receiving enough. If the hands are weak and low energy, they may be taking but not giving back enough.

8

Creating and Activating Sacred Space

'Ike 'ia no ka loea i ke kuahu—
An expert is recognized by the altar they build

The altar or *lele* is used in Hawaiian culture for placing gifts that honor the gods and goddesses, ancestors, and spirits of nature. The Hawaiian proverb above refers to the ability to recognize a master by the integrity with which they build their altar, as an altar signifies the degree of ones' training. It was important to them to offer the proper gifts to specific gods or goddesses in order to please them and receive their blessings. However, this is not the only altar referred to in this proverb.

Take a moment and think about yourself as you sit in your sacred space of existence. In your sacred space—which is you—is the altar of your body, the altar of your mind, and the altar of your spirit. What thoughts do you place in the altar of your mind? What type of substances are you placing on the altar of your body? And finally, what gifts are you offering the altar of your own higher self? How do you honor your spirit? It is important to only place the very best gifts on your altar, honor what you know to be true, and reflect the pristine beauty of the divine within you.

In this chapter, we discuss assembling the Healing Temple, which also includes preparing your body, mind, and spirit for a healing session. When you prepare yourself and the temple space with care and intention, you vibrate at a level of mastery, and more mana (spiritual power) can flow through you!

We call this space a temple because it is a holy space, created and used for communion with ke Akua in service to aloha light for the maturing of consciousness within every human soul here on earth. When a sacred space is created and activated, it is quite humbling to witness the transformations that take place in ourselves and others who have the courage to heal.

The Room: Create a Sacred Space for Healing

You can create a healing temple anywhere. An aura of divine presence is the by-product of a sanctified healing space. People can feel holiness, an unmistakable vibration of warm inclusiveness, similar to the feeling some people get when entering a cathedral. From a shamanic perspective, a house is a living being that remembers what takes place within its walls. Likewise, a house is forever changed by the healing activities you participate in.

The most important ingredients for a healing space are cleanliness, quiet, and warmth. People will come with busy minds, often feeling fragmented. Focus your healing space toward facilitating the stillness of carefully listening to what needs to be brought forward to be resolved, refreshed, or lifted, with minimal distractions. Be creative in making your temple space. Your spirit guides and all the angels are assisting you.

After a healing has happened, there are several methods of cleansing yourself and the energy of the space that are very effective. These may include prayers, smudging, saltwater, aromatherapy, the ringing of bells, beating of drums, sacred music, and shamanic visualizations for transmuting energy. All the different rituals or techniques operate on the principle of makia: *energy flows where attention goes.* Your own sincere intention directs the clearing of the energy through your words, thoughts, and actions. Incorporating some of these techniques into the session will keep the energy moving nicely. After the session, open the doors and windows to let fresh air flow through the room. Vacuum or clean the floors to keep the room fresh and clear.

Gathering Tools and Preparing for a Session

When you decide to create a consecrated space, gathering all the various tools that you want for healing work, it's like a treasure hunt. These tools can assist you in raising the vibrations for you and your receiver to open, surrender, and allow a flow of infinite healing energy. This list covers many of the items we use in our temple. Because we draw from several influences in our healing practice, we use the tools and sacred objects that have meaning to us and those we work with. You can use anything that helps you focus and increase the energy flow, opening to more light, clearing the way for miracles to show up.

Suggested items to support your healing temple:

+ Crystals, wood, or animal totems for the earth element

+ A small bowl of water or shells for the water element

+ Wings and feathers for the air element

+ Incense, smudge, or candles for the fire element

+ Rattles, bells, singing bowls, chimes, or flutes for sound healing

+ Small bowl of Hawaiian alaea salt, flowers, and inspiring pictures

+ Various decks of cards for divination

+ Foot wash tub, chair, tissues, a crystal pitcher with glasses, and drinking water

+ Massage tools, reference books, stereo with music

+ Massage table and massage oil, sheets, two pillowcases and an eye pillow

+ Slippers (for oily feet)

+ A bath towel (for taking a shower after the session)

Building an Altar

The altar is an important focal point, to invoke the life-force within nature for assistance in healing. It is very helpful to acknowledge the nature spirits of fire; water; wind; and stone; and the kingdoms of plant, animal and human. You can use stones, crystals, wood, or animal totems to represent the earth element. Shells, water fountains, or a small bowl of water can be used to represent the water element. Feathers, flutes, or fans can be used to represent the air. A candle, sage, sweet grass, or incense represents the element of fire. You can also place other shamanic healing tools on the altar to be used when needed such as wands, drums, rattles, bells, chimes, singing bowls, sacred oils, herbal offerings, or plant medicines. If you use various decks of cards for divination, these can also be placed on the altar.

In honor of Hawaii, you can place a small bowl of alaea salt upon the altar to acknowledge the presence of the Hawaiian ancestors. It can also be used to draw out/absorb any negative energy being released in the session, especially when placed under the massage table. Another way to honor the Hawaiian ancestors or gods and goddesses is to place a vase of fresh flowers on the altar.

To honor your ancestors or spirit guides, place a picture or a symbol to represent them on the altar. You can place pictures of your loved ones there too. You can place food on the altar to be blessed and energized during the healing session, and then eat it after or offer it to the spirit helpers by placing it outside on the earth. Anything on the altar is blessed and energized by your healing presence and prayers. As most sessions begin with smudging when the receiver enters the room, we always have a smudge stick and/or sweetgrass wand in a fireproof holder on the altar. An eagle or owl feather, or raven wing is used to fan the smudge wand which is lit by the center candle flame that represents the divine fire of the Great Spirit.

Pre-session Protocol

Pre-session protocol serves to align you with the spirits of the building and the land the building stands upon, the various spirits of nature that surround the building, and the spirit of your receiver. These protocols can be the most important thing for the healing to unfold because when a healing takes place, the temple space also receives a healing. If the land or building is harboring spirits of unrest, it may show up in your healing session ... and you may not know where it's coming from.

Before every session, I suggest aligning with your own higher self, your ancestors, and spirit guides, and the higher self, ancestors, and spirit guides of the soul coming to receive the healing. Do it in a quiet, contemplative state with intention. Setting up the space, clearing the energy of the room, lighting a candle on the altar, sitting in meditation to center yourself, and praying to welcome everyone in spirit into the space all serve as forms of opening protocol. Protocols open sacred portals for light to pour in, harmonizing with the spirits in and around your temple.

Opening Prayers

Prayers are the gifts we place on the altar of our heart. If you pray before the client arrives, chances are good you will activate a successful flow of grace throughout the session and after the client leaves. The act of prayer raises your vibration in a powerful way that can be felt by everyone around you. Then people are healed merely by being in your presence.

There are many ways to pray; God has many names. We encourage you to draw from any sources of spirituality that speak to your heart and soul and use whatever form of prayer, song, or chant that works for you for an opening protocol. It is the feeling of profound connection that you get when you chant or pray that alters frequencies!

9

Rituals for the Soul

Ritual has a way of harnessing potent cosmic energy and focusing it for a specific purpose. Here we will share some of the effective rituals that we have developed over the years in honor of the soul and the transformation process. These rituals draw upon influences from many different paths. They can be used individually or incorporated into any type of bodywork session. We encourage you to try them out, or perhaps adapt them into your own healing protocols.

Rituals and ceremonies can open a door to spirit realms, and create a field of intention in the room, around you and the receiver. For any ritual to be effective, we must engage the three souls: body, mind, and spirit. The ku (body) loves to participate in all forms of ritual because it's being stimulated through the physical senses. The deeper the sensory impression on the ku, the more open the body is to engage and offer its support.

Movement builds up energy in the body that can be used for the process of creation. The Iono (mind) takes the energy built up in the body and directs it by using strong words and focused thoughts during each phase of the ritual. When we use a ritual to connect and elevate our consciousness to the level of spirit, transformation takes place because the higher powers (na 'Aumakua) intervene on our behalf here in this physical dimension. Sincere intention is everything in ritual, so a strong opening prayer and a strong ending prayer—both with gratitude—create a powerful container for something wonderful to take place. One of the most powerful aspects of ritual is how it can unify the focus of two or more people together in a common purpose, greatly adding to the power and strength of what you are bringing into form.

Honoring the Soul
Honi, Smudging, Anointing, Bathing the Feet, Affirmative Prayer

Here is an outline of a ritualistic healing session:

+ Welcome the client in with a hug or *honi* when they enter

+ Guide them toward the candle-lit altar to smudge them to clear their aura

+ Anoint them with a sacred oil blend to honor the spirit within their body

+ Bathe and massage their feet in hot water mixed with sea salt and sacred oils

- Address the mental and emotional bodies by opening a truth dialog
- Use a powerful prayer to connect with spirit and set clear intentions for the outcome
- Lead them to the massage table to begin the body-work treatment

As you can see, the combination of all these potent rituals has an impressionable significance on the receiver, greatly enhancing the effect of the massage and the overall bodywork treatment. You can change or adjust any of these rituals to meet an individual's needs by the promptings you feel from the heavenly guidance that is present within you. These blessing rituals feed the souls of both the giver and the receiver on a deep, primal level. They activate ancient memories and elicit assistance from the ancestors and our Creator. The receiver can feel the deep reverence and commitment of the practitioner as they perform these blessing rituals. In this place of trust and safety, they realize they have come to a space where they can surrender fully to release their story, finally letting it go.

The Honi: Greeting the Soul with Aloha

The honi is a traditional Hawaiian protocol, a merging of two souls through a Ha breath. It was used as a gesture among family members or close friends to acknowledge a shared, deep spiritual connection with that person. Today, this is still a common practice of many native Pacific Islanders, and is often used in greeting and parting to show respect. To take part in the act of honi is to share in the Ha—the breath of God by joining forehead to forehead (some look into each other's eyes) and taking a breath together.

Smudging: A Sacred Tradition for Cleansing

Preparation: The practice of smudging—using cedar, sage, or sweetgrass as incense tied together in wands or sticks to burn in a controlled manner—is a blessing and cleansing ritual that can be performed anywhere, anytime, as long as it does not interfere with anyone around you. Choose which type of herbs to use for your smudge. You will need a nonflammable bowl to burn the smudge in as well as a lighter or candle to ignite your smudge. In Hawaii cleansing, blessings are performed using water mixed with alaea salt and a ti leaf. Sometimes turmeric would be added to the water as well. The saltwater is sprinkled over the person or around the room in the same way the smudge is applied.

To begin: When you light the smudge, pray to the spirit of the plant you are burning, and humbly thank it for being with you. Ask it to bring forth its blessing to cleanse, purify, and protect the person, place, or thing you are clearing. This engages the spirit of the plant. These plant medicines are burned and the smoke is wafted over the person, place, or thing that you are blessing.

Cleansing a room: Go around the whole room and waft the smoke into all the corners, doorways, and upper and lower boundaries of the room (smoke can be fanned with your hands or a bird wing or feather that has been blessed).

Cleansing an object: Swirl the burning smudge wand around the object in a circular motion saying a blessing for that object to be purified, blessed, and protected.

Cleansing a person: Begin by fanning the smoke over the front of their body, arms, legs, and head. Have them turn around and do the same on the back of the body.

Pray aloud as you smudge, clear their aura, and wash them in light (and smoke) with respectful inclusiveness. The receiver's eyes are closed, inhaling this blessing, and grounding into the earth, coming fully present. We often use Hawaiian chants, prayers, and songs for blessing. You can use whatever words come to you. A simple smudging prayer would be:

Spirit, purify, bless, and protect this … (whatever it is you are smudging) … !

Repeat this line over and over as you smudge. Be sure to always finish with giving thanks.

Anointing with Oil and Footbath

This ritual builds trust and brings the client into an open-hearted state of relaxation; a deeper surrender. The ritual has five main parts: blessing the water with salt, anointing with oil, bathing and massaging the feet, sharing story and setting intentions, and affirmative prayer.

Preparation: You will need a chair and a large basin for the foot wash. Your receiver will sit in a chair, and you will sit down on the floor in front of the basin at their feet. Fill the basin with hot water and place it on a towel on the floor in front of the chair.

Place about 2 to 4 tablespoons of salt in a little cup or glass, and place it on the floor beside you, next to the basin filled with hot water. Epsom salts work well, but you can also use Hawaiian salt or other natural sea salt, Dead Sea salts, or Himalayan salt.

There are many companies that make unique and lovely essential oil blends, and you can build a small collection of essential oils, using whichever oils that appeal to you. This is a form of plant spirit medicine that can be very fascinating to explore. You can research different companies and also research the healing properties of different plants to create a set of about eight different oils to use for your sacred footbaths. In our halau, we use the Sacred Touch oils, from Bishop Glenda Green's company, Inspired Origination. We love this set of oils because the themes and the fragrances are perfect for this type of ritual. There are eight primary anointing oils in the set; each has a sanctified purpose, blessed by Jeshua (Jesus) and imbued with the potent frequencies of: Abundance, forgiveness, peace, wisdom, joy, compassion, innocence, and Christ scent. If you can't find these oils, look for other companies that make oils with similar themes, or you can create your own.

Take your set of oils and put them in a nice velvet or soft cloth bag so that the receiver can hold it in their lap while waiting to pull an oil blindly out of the bag when prompted. Until then, place the bag of oils on the floor next to the salt, near your cushion across from them and the foot basin.

To begin: Say, "Please have a seat, and place one foot on each side of the tub until we have finished blessing the water." The idea is to have the person sit without placing their feet into the water just yet. Sit on a firm meditation cushion on the floor in front of the tub, facing the receiver after handing them the bag of anointing oils to hold in their lap.

Blessing the Water with Salt

First you will use the salt, calling upon its healing qualities for the benefit of the receiver. Salt has the ability to draw out toxins, negativity, and bitterness.

Pick up your small container (approx. ¼ cup) of salt, hold it over the water basin and say, *'E ho'omaika'i wai keia* (Bless this water). While gradually pouring the salts in a circular motion into the hot water, keep saying *'E ho'omaika'i wai keia,* twice more. Stir with your fingers in the water until the salts are fully dissolved. (No feet in the water basin yet!)

Anointing with Oil—A Sacred Blessing

Now, invite them to reach into the velvet bag and pull out one of the little bottles (without looking in the bag, of course). Invite them to reach into the velvet bag, and pull out one of the little bottles of oil (without looking into the bag, of course). When they hand you one of the bottles of oil, lift it to the sky and use the following words and gestures for blessing their soul cluster. Let's begin with their ancestors. Raise the oil bottle toward the sky and say, "We bless your higher self and all your ancestors." Then hold the oil bottle out in front of you over the basin, toward their head and bless their parent-self, by saying, "We bless the light of your soul that resides within your mind." Now hold the oil bottle over the basin in front of their belly, blessing their child-self saying, "We bless this body with infinite love."

Next open the bottle and turn it upside down with your right hand, waiting for the drops to fall into your open left palm, both hands over the water basin. Allow at least three drops to fall into your left palm, then hold the bottle over the water basin. Allow three more drops to fall into the water saying again, *'E ho'omaika'i wai keia* ("Bless this water").

Now you are ready to anoint the client with the sacred oil of their choosing. Holding the drops of oil in your open palm, take your opposite hand and touch the oil with the tip of your middle finger. Move slowly toward their forehead, saying, "On this day, it is an honor and a blessing to anoint you, beloved brother (or sister) with infinite (use the name of oil chosen by the client)."

Next, using your middle finger again, with a dab of oil, gently, make a small X on their forehead, between their eyebrows (over the pineal gland), then make a circle around the X, enclosing it. Say, "…in your mind." Gently make an X enclosing it with a small circle on the skin over their heart…and say, "…in your heart." Then do the same motion in their palms, one at a time while saying, "...and in your body." Gently make a cross, enclosing it with a small circle in the center of each palm. Finally, a make cross, enclosing it with a small circle in the center, on the bottom of each foot and say, "Everywhere you walk, you will walk with the blessing of ... (insert name of oil)." After anointing each foot, place them into the hot water basin one at a time.

As the person sits with their feet in the water, infuse their being with the healing qualities of the scented oil by having them close their eyes, and bring their open palms together in front of their face, and breathe in deeply, into every cell of their body the aroma of the oil they have just been anointed with—a very potent finish! You can say, "Now bless your soul with the power of (name of oil) by breathing in deeply and offering this gift to every cell of your body!" Have them take at least three deep breaths, inhaling through their nose. This allows the medicinal properties of the essential oils to go directly into the brain. When they finish this, they can relax their hands and lean back into the chair into a deeper presence in their personal environment, infused by the wonderful anointing fragrance, into quiet resolve, integrating this potent moment of aromatic bliss.

Bathing the Feet: An Ancient Honoring of the Soul

People normally pay little or no attention to their feet on a regular basis, so having the feet bathed with loving intention, a healing fragrance, and a deeply healing foot massage is truly heaven for most people. This ancient ritual goes way back; the Bible has accounts of Jesus having his feet washed and anointed by Mary Magdalene. When we anoint someone's feet they may begin to feel their sacred connection to themselves, and feel more grounded on beloved Mother Earth.

Careful Listening

The client must feel absolutely safe and relaxed in your temple for any healing to take place. This ritual will set the stage for allowing their heart to crack open, and if they have anything weighing heavy on their heart that needs to be revealed or expressed, it may come up during these blessing rituals.

While they begin to feel somewhat settled into this peaceful experience, listen very carefully. Some people will be ready to share their feelings and open up immediately; others may require some time or assistance. Relaxing into stillness, begin to massage their feet when you feel it is the perfect moment to do so. This allows their emotional body to settle in and be comforted while some internal rearranging begins to take place in them. After you are promoted to speak, you can assist the person to open up and share what is on their minds by asking a few simple questions:

+ What is the biggest challenge in your life at this time?

+ Are you having any physical challenges at this time? Any pain anywhere?

+ How is your relationship with your ... (parent, loved one, child, or coworker)?

+ Is there anyone you would like to forgive today?

+ Is there some feeling or some pattern you would like to release from your life today?

+ Is there some feeling or quality you would like to bring into your life at this time?

Bone Washing the Feet

Now let's begin to bone wash their feet. Using your fingers (softly at first), feel for and smooth out any lumps of tension with firm but gentle pressure in a spiraling motion using a waltz tempo: *one*-two-three, *one*-two-three. Beginning just below the ankle, clear between all the bones down and out between their toes, then along the bones and out each toe, releasing what no longer belongs. Bone wash around the sides of their heels firmly to include their ankles. Be very attentive to witnessing how the foot massage and the person's heart (revealing its story) affect each other. The foot massage must be gentle enough to allow the person to speak their truth without distracting them from recalling their story but firm enough to create a release.

Acknowledge, Accept, Release

As you work the feet, invite them to keep sharing. Everything that is spoken into this consecrated space is being received by the One Spirit and is being absolved into the highly charged water we have blessed and set before them. Salts absorb energy because they are little crystals from the Earth's belly. Your receiver's story can be completely received and melted away by an undeniable frequency—the presence of absolute, unconditional acceptance. To do this often feels a bit intimidating because the person is revealing things they have never said before to anyone about their feelings and behavior toward others. To be received fully, acknowledged fully, and accepted fully, is the highest form of loving compassion. What it offers to all who are present is so lovely, truly ineffable! We call this the "truth dialog" because it gets to the truth of the matter—the heart of healing—which is to remove what does not belong and to return to our original innocence.

It is important to learn to ask the right questions in the right way, at the right time to get to the root of any issue. A good overall intention you can hold as a facilitator for their session is to reconnect them with their personal power source, to call back their power from wherever they have left it, and to reunite their soul cluster. When we hold on to judgments, fears, and limiting beliefs, we leak our precious mana. Most people have given their power away to other people, places, and things, agencies outside of them like the institutions of marriage, schools, banks, churches, corporations, and governments. Power is also given away to other people: parents, siblings, children, partners, or other relationships. To help the person reclaim mana (personal power) and harness it, encourage them to forgive and release what needs to be let go, and then we ask them to breathe open their heart and reclaim their divine birthright by connecting to their divine light pouring into them from just above their head.

Affirmative Prayer

Finish the session by appealing to a higher power for assistance with the transformation that is taking place. Take the hands of the receiver, and explain to them that it is now time to pray. This way they can be involved in the prayer—fully present. When they are ready, take a deep breath, and begin to pray in your own way, using the information they shared during the footbath for inspiration. After you have shared your part, always ask them if they have anything they would like to add to the prayer. It is empowering for the receiver to pray out loud with you for their own growth and well-being.

Affirmative prayer is an art that anyone can master with enough practice. It affirms the desired state of well-being as already being present in our reality here and now. It works on the principle of *ike*, our thoughts and words create our experience of reality. When you acknowledge the divine that lives within both you and the receiver whole-heartedly, and speak a prayer from this confident yet humble place, the blessing you are calling in will be activated and received within the heart and soul of each of you. We recommend practicing affirmative prayer because it is especially helpful for manifesting a desired state of health and well-being. Here is an example of an affirmative prayer.

> *Divine Creator, we come to you this day in loving humility*
> *with tender open hearts, asking to receive a blessing for*
> (insert name of receiver here). *Thank you for the life*
> *lessons* (insert name) *has experienced as challenges and*

for the healing that's taking place at this time. We know that everything we need to resolve and heal what we've discussed here today, is within us now. We ask your guidance in our thoughts, words, and actions that will bring harmony and cooperation into this situation. We are open to receive what is best for all involved and we bless everyone's part. As we sit here together aligned within divine strength and grace, we claim the blessing of perfect health, perfect peace, and absolute abundance that is everyone's birthright for (insert name).

We know that right here, right now, the blessing of this prayer being answered is entering every part of our awareness, and it is rooting into the center of our body, mind, and spirit as truth. This blessing is now bringing harmony and healing into all our organs, our nervous system, and all other systems within our bodies. Indeed, all areas of our life are brought into alignment for the greater good as we offer and release this prayer. Thank you God for this blessing! And so it is!

Remember to be specific and use the information you were given in the truth dialog to create your prayer. Using affirmative prayer to overcome a big challenge, anger, frustration, and darkness will subside as a shift in awareness toward your inner resources takes place. Your mind will become clear to receive a new perspective or perception, opening a portal for divine intervention. In this form of prayer, you are not praying to anything outside of you, you are praying to the divine that dwells within you and all around you. You are praying in a state of oneness with the divine, and confidently declaring what you know to be true.

Remember that all healing techniques are only that—healing techniques. A good prayer acknowledges each of us as being one with the very source of love. This gives us powerful juice to flow into and through all the techniques. It is the presence of perfection as a god-self within both the giver and the receiver that give the techniques the mana to heal. It is essential for the receiver to express their sincere gratitude before you close the prayer. This is how you can finish this collection of blessings with a strong ending.

Gratitude Prayer

Gratitude prayers carry such powerful loving energy back to our source—the One Spirit. When someone comes to you with a huge challenge to deal with, try using affirmative prayer with gratitude (as hard as it may seem) to shift where you are being pulled to focus your energy. The important thing is to put your sincere feeling into the words. Gratitude helps facilitate a return to the center of the river, where the current of love can carry you both home. Use any words of thanks in your prayer that work for you; the receiver can also add in what they are grateful for too, as this is a very important opportunity for them!

After the prayer and these blessing rituals are complete, the transformation is activated and will continue opening as you begin to perform the shamanic bodywork.

10

Lomilomi Techniques

In this chapter we will share a few basic lomi techniques from our various teachers using hands and forearms that can be applied to many different parts of the body. We will share light touch healing techniques, such as Kahi Loa, bone washing, and other sacred shamanic healing rituals developed by us that work on the level of the soul and the spirit as well as the body. We will also introduce some strokes that can apply deep pressure that also feel very relaxing.

A tremendous amount of mana can flow through the heart and hands of a lomi giver. After doing lomilomi for a few years, your hands will begin to glow. It's true. They actually begin to radiate with so much aloha light that they take on this kind of glowing, pulsating aura of charismatic healing warmth, radiant with unconditional love. Your sacred heart and your healing hands become one in service to aloha. Take the best care of your hands, for they are precious extensions of your sacred heart, creating deep peace for a human race in dire need of this at this time. Bless your amazing healing hands, and let the blessings flow. The gifts you will bring forth through your hands are precious beyond measure.

Serge King's Kahi Loa (Eternal Oneness)

Kahi Loa is a pure form of Hawaiian shamanic healing developed by Serge Kahili King. As Dr. King explains in his book *Instant Healing:* "For me it began with my Hawaiian aunty when I was in my early twenties … What she did was so soft and gentle and simple that I never thought of it as massage for quite some time … I took everything I learned from her, added more things I learned piecemeal from my Hawaiian uncle, and organized it into the system I call Kahi Loa."

Kahi Loa's light touch, energy healing technique calls in and engages the elements of nature for the benefit of the receiver. The practitioner guides the receiver on a meditative, interactive healing journey, contemplating and communing with fire, water, wind, and stone, medicinal plants, healing crystals, power animals, and human spirit beings.

Gentle hand movements are used on the whole body, moving from the head down to the feet to relax the receiver while the giver removes stagnant energy from their body. Kahi Loa uses a shared intention between the giver and receiver, now fully participating in their own healing while receiving a gentle skin massage and shamanic healing.

In Kahi Loa you can use sound, vibration, color, visualization, symbols, humming, and words to enhance the effect of this form of sublime yet profound bodywork medicine. Because it is done through the clothing without oil, it is enjoyable for both young and old and can be performed anywhere. Even plants and animals are receptive to this form of Hawaiian medicine. We invite you to explore these shamanic techniques. All the gifts of nature are waiting here to serve you.

Elements, Elementals, and Kingdoms: The Spirits of Nature

Kahi Loa takes the receiver on a guided journey that allows for them to connect to the spirits associated with each element. To a shaman, the world is inhabited by many, many spirits. Elemental beings are the nature spirits who co-create earthly life forms. Dwelling in all forms of nature, they can be of assistance to all of us. In other cultures, they are called devas, fairies, fauns, gnomes, and elves to name just a handful. We need to be able to open to the possibility that there may be more to life than meets the eye. Perhaps these beings play an equally powerful and important role in our existence. If we disrespect the delicate balance and order of nature, these elemental energies can create imbalances and disease ("dis-ease") in our bodies and our environment. Respecting and acknowledging these powerful elements and kingdoms of nature creates a harmonious cooperation in our growth, abundance, and well-being.

In a deep Kahi Loa session, you allow the spirit within each element—fire, water, wind (air), and stone (earth)—as well as the spirits within the kingdoms of nature—plant, animal, and human—to activate healing in the body, effecting a harmonious, peaceful resolution to take place.

Shamanic Journey

In a shamanic journey, you relax, close your eyes, and use your imagination to create a dream of your own design. This process creates healing on the subconscious level. The process is facilitated by a guide who leads the person through the journey. The guide speaks to the receiver in a calming way, creating the framework for a scene or a desired outcome to take place. The weaving of the story takes the receiver into a healing place within their mind, where they can make prominent changes within their sacred garden. The guide creates a situation for healing, but at the same time, allows them to choose certain parts of the story for themselves, by drawing on the images and ideas from their own sub-conscious mind. In this way, the receiver can be directly connected and actively participating in healing themselves.

In Kahi Loa, we take the receiver on a journey where they can connect to each element and kingdom of nature, and open and receive many healing blessings along the way. Never underestimate your power as a healer to influence reality in this dimension. The cells will often drink in the energy medicine from the particular spirit that you and your receiver have called in. In the raising of their vibration, the subconscious body-mind will just let go of whatever pattern is no longer useful, replacing it with a higher choice.

A kahuna understands and masters the power of *kahea* "to sound the call," which is key to Hawaiian shamanism. Kahea involves understanding your body/mind/spirit soul cluster and how to unite them so they are all involved when you speak. Choose your words carefully and combine them with a vibration that can be directed to bring immediate results. When you master using your voice in healing work, you can take the session to a higher level by speaking (or humming or singing) directly to the subconscious mind of the receiver. In Kahi Loa, your voice guides the receiver into a trance state of wholeness. Every cell has memory of its own perfection and the perfect wholeness of an integrated system within the body. As a giver, to call in and affirm this perfection of wholeness activates the memory within the cells.

Quantum physics proves to us that the tiny subatomic particles that make up all life are telepathically aware. Conscious and always changing, they respond to our attention and intention. Ancient Hawaiians knew this and could communicate with these particles in nature, such as influencing the weather by communing with a storm to bring it into a peaceful resolve. In ancient times, the kahuna healed broken bones by communicating with the cells within the broken bone and encouraging them to knit back together. There was a saying: *He pu'upa hiolo wale no i ka leo*, "an obstructing wall falls down at the sound of the voice."

The voice is powerful. Used properly, it can instigate great change. In Kahi Loa, the receiver uses their voice to sound their intentions and take responsibility for their healing process. The giver's gentle voice accompanies the techniques being used on the body. The receiver chooses stones, plants, animals, and human spirits to help with their healing process and communicates to the giver what they are feeling in their body as changes occur along the way.

Serge King's Kahi Loa Technique

Preparation: The receiver lies on a bed or massage table. They can wear light, loose clothing. If they like, they can use a sheet over their body. In a full Kahi Loa session, we call to the spirit of each element, and then call to each of the kingdoms of nature. However, you can use any one of these techniques anywhere, anytime. We usually begin with the receiver lying facedown, and do all the elements and the plant and animal kingdoms. Then we have them turn over and we do the movements for all the elements again and the plant, animal, and finish with the human kingdom.

To begin: Tell the receiver you are leading them on a healing journey, connecting with the spirits of nature, beginning with the elements.

Tell the receiver that you will begin by calling in the spirit of fire and then ask them, "When you think of fire, what type of fire comes to your mind? What color is it? What qualities does it have?" Then you will invoke the spirit of fire by saying, "Kahi Ahi" and apply the technique for fire.

After they have a clear image of fire in mind, call in the spirit of fire and apply the fire technique.

Begin at the top of the head with the bodywork. Moving down the body, communicate directly with the cells, which will reconfigure in accordance with your loving intention. Use your words to re-enforce the qualities of fire the person has chosen. It is not a forceful command, but rather a call to remembrance of harmony, wholeness, and peace. The elements and kingdoms of nature exist inside the human body, and can be summoned and brought into alignment with healing intentions. Use your breath to move the energy and clear the body of any stuck or dense areas as you work.

After you have finished going down both sides of the body with fire, you can announce that it's time to call-in the spirit of water. Have them visualize any type of water that comes to mind. Then you will invoke the spirit of water by saying "Kahi Wai", and apply the next technique, and so on.

There is a specific type of hand movement associated with each element that is applied to the body of the receiver as the practitioner moves through the various segments of the session. At the beginning of each segment, have the client choose an image to focus on each time. The idea is to use the first image that pops into their mind. When they call in the spirit of something without forethought, they are choosing their own perfect energetic medicine. Have the person visualize each element in their mind and also share what they are feeling as they meditate on the qualities they associate with that particular plant, animal, or whatever they are calling into their healing.

The elements: *Ahi* (fire) uses a raking hand/finger motion, with finger tips and nails; *Wai* (water) uses a gentle, yet firm pressure, washing motion with all the pads of the hands and fingers, flowing over the body like, clear, running water; *Makani* (wind) uses no physical touch, with open palms to clear the magnetic field, three inches above the skin over the whole body; *Pohaku* (stone) uses still hands (no movement) with a firm touch, often with humming.

When you are ready to call to the spirit of stone, ask the receiver to pick a specific crystal or rock for their healing, again asking them what it signifies to them. Then the giver invokes the spirit of that specific crystal, "Kahi Pohaku", calling in its healing qualities into various parts of the body that require this kind of medicine.

After sharing each of these elemental modules, the practitioner calls on the three kingdoms of nature. The receiver picks a particular plant, a particular animal, and finally a human spirit for their healing.

La'au (plant) uses the sides of the hands, alternating hand over hand in a circular motion, with relaxed, soft fingers brushing down the body with a brisk tempo, and a rolling "watermill" tempo. *Holoholona* (animal) uses open hands with a deep, penetrating, slow squeezing, twisting, and kneading of the muscles. *Kanaka* (human) uses light touch with a few fingerpads, connecting the chakras, and leapfrogging down the chakras and then the major joints of the body. If you really want to have a powerful finish to your Kahi Loa session, refer to the Kanaka process outlined in chapter 11, in the Kaulike section of the Golden Cocoon activation.

Harry Uhane Jim's Traditional Hawaiian Touch Medicine

Harry Uhane Jim was born and raised in the small Hawaiian village of Anahola on Kauai before moving to the Big Island in his adult life. He learned many things about healing and energy from daily occurrences with various powerful members of the family and the community. Uncle Harry embodies the spirit of aloha and shares it generously in a Hawaiian style way. He speaks the secrets as a pure channel for the Hawaiian ancestors and his own spirit guides. He serves as a uniting, inclusive force that gathers light workers into sacred circle. He reminds us that we can all be agents of change, in service to the light, and through his traditional bodywork techniques he helps us to anchor joy here on earth.

Many people find Uncle Harry's teachings refreshing because Harry shows us that healing can be easy and fun. Harry teaches grassroots healing in a true Hawaiian way. He's distilled thirty years of learning and practicing lomilomi into what he calls Hawaiian Touch Medicine, and he shares it as five simple techniques that in Harry's own words, are done with "easy aloha."

Some of the bodywork techniques we have learned from Uncle Harry include:

+ *Creating space*: Creating space between the bones and joints of the body through the use of lifting, wiggling, shaking, pulling, and pounding in connection with breathing fully and deeply to release stuck energy as the client breathes deeply.

+ *Bone washing:* Cleaning and clearing the skin on the bones, removing density or crystallized energies from the joints out to the extremities.

+ *Po'o:* Bone washing techniques are used for clearing all the bones of the head and face.

+ *Ha breath medicine:* Uses the breath of life to transmute and clear stuck emotion and "expired contracts" with self and others.

+ *Laulima:* The practice of laying on of hands, often performed in a group.

Uncle Harry shares what he's gathered in his life with others in a joyous and humorous way. In his teachings, Harry takes us out of our small thinking mind or small selves and into our greatness, offering us a way to become big enough to envelop and resolve any problem with easy aloha. He offers a viewpoint of spiritual sovereignty in which one can release themselves from a place of victimhood at the mercy of family and world dramas, and begin to feel themselves at the center of their universe as an empowered, confident, abundant, radiant being.

He teaches us that without forgiveness, healing cannot be fulfilled. His famous phrase to all his students is: "There are only two kinds of forgiveness—now or later!"

Uncle Harry draws from the teachings of Daddy Bray, a powerful and well-known kahuna who left behind a very profound legacy that still lives on today. Here is a quote from Daddy Bray's book, *Kahuna Religion of Hawaii*:

> Christ taught the Kingdom of God is within us. What does this mean? The kahunas teach the same thing! Within us are both Spirit and Matter. We must know both of them. All the ways the kahuna had to heal, to control nature, to bless and to curse are based on this one secret. Reality is the true, error is the unreal. How can you replace error with the Real? We have to reflect the light of God and stop fearing the darkness. Even if a person is weak he can be sincere in his efforts to overcome fear. If he is sincere God will send invisible helpers to give strength and destroy the dark forces. Gradually confidence will replace doubt. Love will replace fear.

As a contemporary kahuna, Uncle Harry includes many influences in his teachings and invocations. He is a channel for spirit and shares life-changing messages with his students while elevating them with the kahuna transmission.

> *My job isn't to give you a list that you can read later.*
> *My job is to ignite the spark of light that lives in you.*
> —Uncle Harry

Harry Uhane Jim's
Bone Washing Technique

"Before clock time began, the Hawaiian healer saw the periosteum (the skin of the human bone) as the cache where memory of physical movement, memory of painful emotions, and memory of abuse lurk. These memories store up one after another like rocks that eventually become mountains. But those memories can also be brought to the surface and released through hands on healing called Bone Washing."—Harry Uhane Jim, *Wise Secrets of Aloha.*

The clearing of the bones can be a light relaxing experience, or it can go to a deeper level when applied in a shamanic way. This technique can release memories of past lives, while clearing the *pilikia* (karma) of the entire family lineage. It can be done with light pressure or with deep, intense pressure. The key is to tune in to the script. What is the body calling for? A light pressure, medium pressure, or deep pressure can all be effective at different times for different people. You can always ask for feedback from the person you are working on.

Preparation: The receiver lies on a bed or massage table. They can wear light, loose clothing. If they like, they can use a sheet over their body.

To begin: Have the receiver lie on their back, and place your fingertips on their sternum. Uncle Harry teaches to use the fingertips, beginning at the center of the body at the chest or sternum, moving outward along the edges of the bones. Your fingers are doing a waltz-style rhythm: *one*-two-three, *one*-two-three going in a small spiraling motion along the bones out to the chest, into the bones of the shoulders, down the arms, and out the hands.

Apply the same technique moving along the edges of the rib bones, down into the pelvis and the hips, then down the legs and out the feet.

Next, reach under the neck and down as far as is comfortable to the vertebrae in between the shoulders and move up the neck, one vertebrae at a time, and up to the head. Touch and remove any stagnant energy from every part of the skull and face. You can work with the energy to move and release what does not belong, by breathing love into each part of the head as you wash the bones moving in little spirals with a one-two-three rhythm. Silently hold a space of acceptance and care, feeling the energy shift as you gently work along the edges of the bones. See if you can feel any blockages or changes in the energy as you work. Encourage the receiver to breathe and be aware of what they are feeling. Encourage the receiver to breathe and stay aware of what they are feeling, while guilding the energies to move out the extremities.

Aunty Margaret's Big Island Massage

Perhaps the most well-known teacher of lomi is Aunty Margaret Machado from the Big Island. No book on lomi would be complete without an honorable mention of this beloved kumu. Her teaching was holistic in its approach, combining colon cleansing with saltwater from the ocean, herbs, and steam baths, as well as breathwork, ho'oponopono, and massage.

She was one of the first native Hawaiians to share the teachings of lomi openly. Aunty Margaret bridged the old Hawaiian ways and those of the modern world; bringing lomi into the realm of massage therapy. To train with Aunty, a student was required to reside with her for at least a month. In addition to their classes on massage, they would cleanse their colon, have regular steam baths and do daily ho'oponopono by the ocean. During this time, the student would be able to heal themselves, witness and participate in the healing of others, and grasp some of the deeper spiritual concepts that a lomi giver needs to succeed.

The lomi of the Big Island is therapeutic and nurturing. There are specific moves to pinpoint specific muscle groups, and also to flush out and pump fresh blood through the body. Different massage moves flow over the body in a dance-like rhythm, many of them resembling the waves of the ocean. We introduce the Ocean Wave stroke in the technique section that follows. There was a lot of focus given to working the belly, and moving what doesn't belong through ho'oponopono—releasing unforgiven memories and trauma stored in the tissues.

Though Aunty taught many techniques in this style of massage, the use of prayer, faith, and love for healing were at the forefront of all her teaching. She was known for being an extremely intuitive and gifted healer. She was very clever and perceptive, and she could tell many things about a person just from looking at them. When Aunty Margaret was asked how she performed miraculous healings on the massage table, she used to say, "Lomilomi is a praying work. I just love the person—God does the rest!" Over the years, a great many people learned lomilomi from Aunty at her little beach house on the Kona coast of the Big Island, Hawaii. One of her many students was Harry Uhane Jim.

Aunty Margaret's Big Island Lomi Technique

Ocean Wave Stroke

Many of the strokes used in Aunty Margaret's style of lomi from the Big Island resemble waves washing upon the shore. The ocean wave strokes are applied in sets of threes: the first wave being the shortest, the second being a little longer, and the third wave being the longest. This pattern of three strokes is typically repeated three times. This type of lomi stroke can be applied to any limb of the body, such as the arms, legs, or the upper back. We will demonstrate it on one side of the back of the body here. Using full soft hands, apply this stroke in a flowing rhythm, as a warm-up stroke with light to medium pressure, with lots of breath and love.

Preparation: Have your massage oil handy for application. The receiver lies facedown on a massage table. This is best applied with the receiver wearing no clothing at all. Use a sheet to drape over private areas and expose only the areas you are massaging (in this case we undrape one whole side of the body). Oil the side of the body with reverence and love.

To begin: Once the oil is evenly distributed, you may begin the ocean wave stroke. Glide from the ankle up to the knee, and caress back down to the ankle. Glide from the ankle, up to the hip or just above the hip, and then caress back down. Glide from the ankle all the way up and over the shoulder and caress down the whole side of the body. Repeat these sets of three waves over and over until the body is warmed up and relaxed.

Sherman Dudoit's Heartworks: Traditional Old Style Lomilomi

This style of lomi came from a powerful kahuna on Maui, and was brought to the world by Sherman Dudoit. This "old style" lomi was part of a bone-setting tradition. In ancient times, the Hawaiians used very crude weapons in battle. Combined with their martial art, called Lua, they would dislocate joints, tear flesh, and break bones on impact; warriors came back from battle in need of much care. This form of traditional Hawaiian massage was implemented to increase circulation, soften the muscles and prepare the body for bone setting (chiropractic-style adjustments).

Sherman was chosen by his kumu in the traditional apprenticeship style, in which the teacher chose only one student to pass the blessing of their teachings on to. Sherman went to see his kumu every day at his home, and trained with him one-on-one, until his training was *pau* (complete). Sherman was taught Hawaiian structural alignment techniques by his kumu, who was skilled in the art of bone setting. Sherman would assess where the misalignment was in the structure of his clients, and then performed specific chiropractic-style adjustments during the lomilomi massage.

Much to his surprise, Sherman was told by his teacher during his training that he would be sharing and teaching this style of lomi all over the world. It was Sherman's kumu who decided on the name "Heartworks" for this type of lomi to be carried into the world because the work comes from and through the heart. He was taught to be careful not to change any part of what he had been taught, and to pass the teaching on to others exactly how it was taught to him. This is the meaning of tradition.

After his training was complete, Sherman was not contacted again by his kumu until right before his passing. When this time came, Sherman returned to Hawaii to the kahuna's bedside. At that time, he was called in so that his kumu could pass on a blessing to Sherman before his body was laid to rest. The Hawaiian practice called "passing on the blessing" refers to breathing a Ha breath into the body of their chosen *haumana* (student) to impart their mana and an energetic transmission of the medicine they carry. In this way, the teacher lives on through that student and the tradition is perpetuated. As he lay dying, the kahuna passed on his last blessing through his breath to Sherman of this ancient lineage, and that is when Sherman's training was complete—he became kumu.

Sherman Dudoit's Non-Dual Approach to Healing

Sherman's approach to lomi was reverent and meditative. His spiritual training centered around meditation, spending much time in silence. These teachings were called Advaita, or Non-dualism. Non-dualism goes beyond genders, the desires and perceptions of the ego mind, the identification with the body—directly into oneness with God. This is the mindset Sherman brought to the table in his lomilomi sessions, pure communion with the divine.

The Heartworks Technique

The basis of each Heartworks session is to be a gift of aloha which comes from a pure, open heart. The heart center is called *pu'uwai*. *Pu'u* means a mound or a hill, and *wai* means fresh water, or blood. Lomilomi is truly a heart-centered form of healing, and there is a particular way it works into a Heartworks session. Much attention is placed on breathing divine light and love in from above, through the top of our head, which Sherman called "the mouth of God" into our heart and out through our hands as we lomi the body. We have come to call this technique the "waterfall of aloha."

EXERCISE: Waterfall of Aloha

Sherman was taught that the crown chakra, the top of the head is the "mouth of God," where we can invite the holy Ha breath to enter and flow through our heart and out our hands onto the one before us on the massage altar. This meditation can also be used as a personal clearing in a ho'oponopono process. The light you draw in from above can clear the lower energies and emotional attachments of fear, judgment, and limitation held in the body, raising and transmuting those energies into pure divine light.

Connect with your higher self. Ask for its power to wash down over you with the light of aloha as an unconditional waterfall of divine love. Visualize standing in a radiant waterfall of light pouring onto you, washing through you as you breathe it in from above. Inhale aloha light cascading from above, into and through your heart. Exhale the light of aloha from your heart down your arms, into your hands, extending this liquid intimacy to envelop yourself (or the person before you) in compassion.

In a Heartworks session, the giver is directing this waterfall of Aloha through their head, their heart and out their hands as they work. The client feels their body, mind, and spirit being cleansed with waves of infinite love.

Sherman Dudoit's Heartworks Technique

The use of hands was preferred by Sherman's kumu and was believed to hold more mana than the forearms. The massage was all about increasing circulation of the blood and flushing the lymphatic fluids within various muscle groups, releasing tension with aloha. The flowing strokes bring new fresh blood into the muscles, which oxygenates the cells and sends healing nutrients into the organs of the body.

Preparation: Have your massage oil handy for application. The receiver lies facedown on a massage table. This is best applied with the receiver wearing no clothing at all. Use a sheet to drape their body, covering private areas and exposing the areas you are massaging. In this case, we undrape one whole side of the body. Oil the side of the body with reverence and love.

To begin: Once the oil is evenly distributed, you may begin the alternating stroke.

Alternating Stroke up the Body

This stroke uses full hands, fingers slightly splayed, and a repetitive alternating motion, hand over hand, moving up the belly of the muscle, repeating over and over using a brisk tempo. This kind of traditional lomi is very repetitive and rhythmic, creating a trance for reducing tension in the muscles. You do not move up to the next section of the body until the part of the limb you are working on is warmed up and flushed.

- Begin at the ankle, full hands alternating with firm pressure, moving upward, from ankle to knee.

- Full hands alternating upward strokes with firm pressure, from knee up the back of the thigh.

- Full hands alternating upward strokes with firm pressure, into buttock and hip area.

- Full hands alternating upward strokes with firm pressure, from hip up side of back and down the arm.

Alternating Stroke down the Body

Glide up the arm and position yourself at the head of the table and begin the alternating stroke going down the body in the following sections:

- Top of shoulder, down one side of the spine
- Down buttock
- Down thigh to knee
- Down the calf, knee to ankle

After warming up the back of the body with these firm pressure strokes, you can then begin to apply an even deeper pressure, using Dancing Thumbs and the Long Stroke from the ankle, up the body, around the shoulder, to the fingertips, and back.

Temple Style Lomi

Kahu Abraham's Kahuna Bodywork—Temple Style Lomi
One lineage of lomi that surfaced in the 1980s and has become widely adapted into the Western culture is Temple Style lomi, which is also called Kahuna Bodywork. Its popularity stems from its unique blend of traditional and contemporary approaches to healing. It is taught as a massage/dance that offers spiritual intimacy through heightened trance states of consciousness to expand into for creating permanent changes in your body and in your life. It is a sensuous, creative, and free-flowing experience. The man who brought Kahuna Bodywork into the world is Kahu Abraham Kawai'i

Abraham was born in 1939, in Ho'okena, on the Kona Coast of the Big Island. At that time it was forbidden to speak Hawaiian, let alone aspire to become a kahuna. However, his gifts were recognized at a young age and he gravitated to individuals who connected him to the wisdom of the kahuna. Later in life, Abraham's kahuna training would bring him to the arts of hula *kahiko* (ancient story-telling dance) and lua (Hawaiian martial arts). He became skilled at navigation, geomancy, and healing, all playing into his presentation to the world and the bodywork he developed, practiced, and taught.

As Abraham traveled and taught his way of sacred alignment, controversy grew. He did not live by the protocols of his peers or the morals of society at large. In breaking away from the traditional training he received, he developed a style of Hawaiian shamanic bodywork that was revolutionary and uniquely his own; one that would profoundly alter the lives of many. With a radical and adventurous approach to life, Abraham would lead his students through deeper and deeper levels of initiatory discovery to grow and strengthen their personal power and spiritual connection within their space of existence. In short, by presenting challenges for others to overcome, he assisted them to find and build their core strength as well as accessing a deeper connection to the stars—transforming their inner game as a spiritual warrior.

Kahu's primary gift was alignment through intimate, cosmic communion using a nontraditional contemporary art form called Temple Style. The phrase "Temple Style" implies that each healing is a sacred ceremony—similar to an ancient rite of passage that was performed in the temples of old. The distinguishing features of Kahuna Bodywork are:

- Flowing forearm strokes that are creative, dynamic, and rhythmic.

- Sacred geometric patterns are used in a massage/
  dance that unlocks and unblocks energy, realigns it
  with its true purpose, and sets it free.

- Following the script of your receiver's body/mind
  from moment to moment rather than a set traditional
  routine or massage therapy routine.

- Deep, surgical strength joint rotations on the arms
  and legs, clearing and opening the shoulders, hips,
  knees, elbows, ankles, and wrists.

- *Ka'aleleau* (the flight) shamanic trance/dance for cosmic alignment, expansion, opening portals, and clearing a pathway for transformational healing in both
  the giver and receiver.

The term "Temple Style" was derived from a video/lecture in Los Angeles recorded December 9, 1987, where Abraham introduced his work to the public. He spoke about his demonstration of a few temple styles that would follow a script:

"The higher self of the person receiving the lomilomi has contracted you, the dancer, to perform the routine and read their body as the script. You must learn to read their body as a dancer reads a script, and follow their body's direction as you perform the lomilomi."

Kahu carried a very specific kahuna wave never seen or felt before. He knew how to enliven the cells, using what he calls "the breath that aligns the breath," in such a way as to bring them into a deeper experience of healing. This served beautifully to awaken the sleeping, sluggish, or blocked energy in the physical body, mind, and also within the deeper realms of the infinite soul. New patterns of flow opened up within the receiver. Lifetimes of expired baggage were cleared. The receiver was often left speechless, feeling empty, and wondering what had happened.

Although Kahu Abraham trained several teachers, many students took what they learned from him and felt called to practice and teach on their own. Each one developed their own style, flavor, and presentation of Kahu's work.

> When you touch another with aloha, it is a merging of
> souls into light. "You" disappear, and so does the "other."
> The bodies melt into a luxurious, luminescent oneness.
> You are then on a soul journey with that person,
> swimming through a sea of energy that is the Universe
> of the other, removing that which does not belong.
> With healing waves of aloha cascading through you
> both, you bear witness to the process of recovering that
> which is the absolute truth of their being—wholeness,
> wellness, innocence, and freedom.—Kealohi

This is all taking place within the context of a thorough, transformative massage with assisted stretching and shamanic bodywork. Here are some of the basic components of what has come to be known as Temple Style lomi or Kahuna Bodywork.

Abraham Kawai'i's
Temple Style Lomi Techniques

Forearm Strokes for Back

When we share Temple style lomi, we find it helpful to employ the navigational terms used in sailing for teaching the deepest strokes. When you navigate a boat into shallow water, you want to avoid the coral reefs as you enter various channels. It is the same when doing massage, using your forearms and elbows as a massage tool. You can think of all the bones (the scapula, hips, sacrum, and spine) as the reefs, and your forearm and elbow as the keel of the boat, navigating through the channels, steering clear of reefs while using a deeper pressure application. It is very important to remain aware of how your elbow is like the keel of a boat. One must be very careful to navigate around and through the reefs with the utmost precaution, attentive awareness, and sensitivity.

Transformational Bodywork Strokes

Temple style massage is performed primarily using the forearms as the pressuring tool along with some deep channel clearing using the elbows. We suggest you use the widest part of your forearm—about an inch and a half from the elbow, as the primary pressuring "tool" for this style of bodywork. In our halau we call this tool your power pad.

In Kahuna bodywork, the forearm and elbow are used to reorganize the energetic flow of the body's matrix, opening clear channels of vital energy along with all the primary energy portals of your being so that more light can enter. Using the forearms and elbows in this way tends to save the lomi giver's wrists and hands from compression injury. These forearm strokes can be done all the way up and down the body while dancing, using a variety of different speeds and varying pressures, while utilizing different types of breathing to create frequencies that reform cellular memory within the organs of the body. Many receivers have stated that they experienced a feeling of ocean waves, or water flowing over and through their entire body.

In this type of bodywork, the practitioner learns how to navigate their dance, following the script, running geometrical patterns of pressure and release on the upper back, moving the energy up and down the spine, as well as pulling it back up the sides of the rib cage with open hands, up from their hips to under the arms, up over their back toward the center of their chest, and finally up the neck to the cranium.

The alternating left and right figure-eight pattern over their heart opens the "rear" heart chakra, and balances the masculine and feminine sides of the body and brain. When their mind begins to let go, surrendering to the pleasurable sensations, the stuck energy and the tension will also let go and flow downstream and out the extremities.

Preparation: The receiver lies facedown on a massage table. This is best applied with the receiver wearing no clothing at all. Use a sheet to drape their body, covering private areas and exposing the areas you are massaging. Have your massage oil handy for application. Oil the back of the body with reverence and love.

To begin: Once the oil is evenly distributed, you may begin the forearm strokes.

Forearm Strokes for Back

Begin with your fingertips at the trapezius, and glide into the trapezius, gradually increasing the pressure as you lean into the trapezius with your forearm.

Glide up with your forearm vertically alongside the spine and press firmly into the space around the shoulder blade.

Three-Quarter Stroke

Turn your arm and your body, positioning yourself horizontally on the side of the body, and press firmly around the scapula, and then down the side of the back toward the hips with your forearm.

When your forearm lands at the sacrum, slide down the hip bone toward the table; switching to hands, caress back up the side of the body, toward the shoulders, and begin the same stroke on the other side of the body beginning at the trapezius

Full Stroke

For the full stroke, when you arrive at the hip/sacrum area with your power pad, you slide down the hip, and then glide up on an angle, into the buttock, and press and lean your forearm into the gluteus maximus.

Spinal Irrigation

The same stroke can be performed with both arms/elbows, creating a deep spinal irrigation. Begin at the trapezius, and press and lean power pads into the traps with both forearms, and then press firmly into the space between the shoulder blades and up the spine and deeply press down both sides of the spine with your elbows, into the spinal processes, until you get to the hip/sacrum area, and then glide down, opening your arms, sliding off the hips, spreading your hands open, caressing back up the sides of the rib cage to the shoulders.

Forearm Strokes on Legs

Deep forearm strokes can be applied to the backs of the legs, beginning at the ankle and sinking into the back and side of the calves, and then the back and side of the thighs.

Deep Release Joint Rotations

Temple style lomi also can involve deep joint rotations incorporated with the massage. Joint rotations can offer healing medicine for releasing issues being held within the joints—undefined, unforgiven, crystalized energy. These rotations offer a "clearing" of emotions that may be trapped in the shoulders, knees, wrists, ankles, hips, and elbows. We work with the ball-and-socket aspect of the joint, addressing what's been held there that does not belong, offering it freedom, to flow into the lymph system. Then with deep tissue massage, we can flush it out. We teach these rotations as a slow-motion meditation.

This allows the receiver's body time to relax under a strong torching pressure using micro-moments. The intention is to clean and clear the joints, offering them more flexibility, as in a frozen shoulder or any other restricted range-of-motion that may be present. When done slowly enough with the utmost care, awareness, and respect, these rotations can be very sensitive yet effective medicine for those who really need their joints cleared of emotional wounds and crystallized energy from unforgiven loved ones, which would include their ancestors.

11

Sacred Rites

Altering the Map within the Brain
Clearing the Past and Future (Prone)

Here is a simple bodywork technique that we developed to remove what does not belong from the head of the receiver—erasing the clutter of busy thoughts from the head to bring the receiver into pa'a (grounded stability).

Preparation: Have your massage oil handy for application. The receiver lies facedown on a massage table. This is best applied with the receiver covered with a sheet, after you have worked on the back of the body, and just before you are about to have them turn over to work on the front of the body. Oil the scalp with reverence and love.

To begin: Remind the receiver that all time is now, and that their infinite potential can be accessed in this moment if they are willing to release themselves from expired contracts and outdated beliefs and obligations.

This is done like shaking an Etch-A-Sketch board upside down. You can visualize this happening with the patterns inside their brain. Using your fingertips as a 'shamanic eraser', with a firm, rapid application, with a rapid, vigorous back-and-forth motion to erase unwanted memories and limiting projections: first, vertical with one hand, then horizontal with the other hand. One hand holds the occipital still while the other does the fast back-and-forth motion. You are thinking of opening new pathways of flow for them, clearing space for new patterns to grow, supporting their infinite potential. This process is amplified when you breathe a waterfall of aloha in through your crown and out through your hands while pouring the light of positive-change into their head (po'o).

Past and Future into Pa'a

In this present moment here and now, we can be free of our story, blessed and blissed, in the center of the current of infinite aloha. In Serge Kahili King's huna teachings, the principle "now is the moment of power" is called *manawa*. In Uncle Harry's halau, "being present" is called *pa'a*. Pa'a refers to a solid foundation, being packed full, or firmly held. It is about being present, connected to all the elements with your attention focused on one task.

In this healing ceremony, we bring the receiver to the point of convergence of time, space, and gravity where the only awareness of self that remains is a "lightness-of-being" love alive. The teachings of a kahuna serve as a reminder that all of our stories are being held in memory—of our past—and because of those memories, we carry limiting projections of false hope, fear, and worry into our future. When we choose to be totally present in the moment, the past is not affecting us because we are not perpetuating habitual memories. In some spiritual circles (as ACIM), these moments are called "holy instants" where pure, cosmic potential for the interaction of spirit (light) and matter (flesh) reside. These are the miracle moments that every healer strives to promote and experience.

This next ritual can be an effective tool for opening to a permanent change, using their will—with a strong proclamation—to enter the current of loving possibilities held within the present moment and to be born anew. It involves clearing various energetic portals on the head and face while stretching and opening the neck and spine.

+ Bone washing the face: Peeling off all previous masks of personas

+ Releasing the past with blessings: Detaching from memories

+ Releasing the future with blessings: Detaching from expectations

+ Declaring to be born anew in every moment

+ Taking the first breath into a new life

Preparation: Have your massage oil handy for application. The receiver lies faceup on a massage table. This is best applied with the receiver wearing no clothing at all. Use a sheet to drape their body, covering the front of their body.

This ritual is very powerful when done on its own, but it was originally created as one of several processes in a several hour healing session. This takes place just after helping the receiver turn over, as a transition into deeper surrender, before working on the front of the body. It is best done with the receiver lying directly on the table, face up, with some oil already underneath them so you can easily slide your hands under their back.

Place a chair at the end of the table, just above their head. Apply a very small amount of oil to their face, lightly tracing the various lines on their face with your fingers, following the bone structure, contours, and muscle fibers.

To begin: Start with bone washing the face. This part of the ceremony symbolizes removing a mask that represents the old story or the egoic personality. We remove the false identities the client is presenting to the world so that their true identity as light can shine through.

1. Placing your fingers under their chin and your thumbs just above the chin, in the center. Press firmly, opening it deeply with the tips of your thumbs, pressing down and out the upper side of the jawbone, moving slowly toward the ears, until your thumbs get to the place where the ear connects to the head. (Do this three times, progressively firmer.)

2. Place the tips of your thumbs above the lips and under the nose, follow the contour of the upper lip pressing down, around, under the cheeks and toward the ears again. (Three times, progressively firmer.)

3. Using your thumb pads again, place them on each side of the nose bridge, at the very top. Massage slowly down both sides of the nose bridge, pressing down around the lower cheeks and toward the ears. (Do this three times, a little firmer each time.)

4. Using your thumb pads again, begin at the same place, on each side of the nose bridge, at the very top. Press slowly down the sides of the nose bridge, clearing just under the cheekbone, finishing at the ears. (Do this three times, getting firmer.)

5. Using your thumb pads again, begin at the very top on each side of the nose bridge. This time, slowly clear along the eye sockets, coming away from the nose bridge and across the top of the cheekbone. (Both sides three times).

6. Turn your thumbs around now, so your thumbnails are pointing away from you and insert them into the upper ridge of the eye sockets on both sides, at the top of the nose bridge, just under the eyebrows. This time, apply a medium pressure, pushing with your thumb pads into the "upper rim" of the eye socket, bone washing from the nose bridge, under the eye brow, outward toward the ear. (Do this three times.)

7. Clear the forehead of tension and open the "third eye" to receive and transmit more light. Beginning with your thumbs pointing away from you, side by side,

pointing toward their nose, press into the forehead and slowly open the area just above their eyebrows outward from the center. Do this three times (lower, middle, and top of forehead), finishing each stroke at the place where the ear attaches to the skull.

Remove your hands from the body of the receiver in between each segment of the ritual, and you will have a greater effect when you touch them again. In the next phase of this ritual, you assist the receiver to erase their attachments to the past and the future.

We lead the receiver in a three-breath rhythm doing three segments with three deep breaths each time, and then one final breath (very deep and long); altogether it is ten breaths. Three for the past (clearing the left side of the face), three for the future (clearing the right side of the face), and three for the present, (clearing both sides of the face). Finally, we do one long inhale and exhale as we clear the spine and stretch the head.

Clearing the Past and Future— Opening to the Present

Part One: Erasing the Past

Say: "Please repeat after me:'I release the past with my blessing!'" The receiver says, "I release the past with my blessing!" You say, "Take three deep breaths and make it so!"

With their first breath, slide your right hand, open, palm up under their neck, cradling their head in your palm. With their second breath, turn their head slightly to the right. On their third breath and final exhale, bring the fleshy part of your left forearm into contact with their forehead and gently swipe your inner forearm one time down the side of their face. (Careful: do not apply any pressure on their eyeball!) At the end of that forearm stroke, glide your left hand up across the top of the shoulder and then under the back of the neck and squeeze up the back of their head, pulling the past right out of the back of their head. Pull the energy of the past out of the head and throw it behind you using the power of your intention. Now you will repeat this segment on the right side of the face, releasing attachments to their future.

Part Two: Erasing the Future

Say: "Please repeat after me: 'I release the future with my blessing!'" They respond, "I release the future with my blessing!" You then say, "Now take three deep breaths, and make it so!"

On their first breath, gently slide your left hand, palm up, under their neck and cradle the head. On the second breath, turn their head slightly to the left. On their third breath and final exhale, bring the fleshy part of your right forearm into contact with their forehead and gently swipe your inner forearm one time down the side of their face. Slide your right hand under their skull, gently squeezing as you comb the future out of their mind. Pull the energy of the future out of the head and throw it behind you!

With the memories of the past and projections of the future out of the way, we can view every moment as new, unbridled from attachments to the past or future! In this next segment, you will take the receiver through a symbolic birthing process.

The next combination of moves metaphorically symbolizes coming through the birth canal, being reborn into the world anew. It can be an initiation of the soul. In this light, you as the lomi giver are a midwife for their soul's renewal.

Part Three: Opening the Present

Say: "Repeat after me, if you would please. (Speak very clearly with confidence, as a proclamation.) 'I choose to be born in every moment new!'" They say, "I choose to be born in every moment new!" After this, you say, "Now take three deep breaths, and make it so!"

On their first breath, stand up. On their second breath, lift your arms high above their chest with your palms facing upward ready to receive their gift of *mana* from above. On their third and final breath, bring both your forearms together above their face, keeping the birthing process in your awareness as they inhale. As they are exhaling you say, "When this last breath is fully exhaled, hold your breath out."

As they exhale, bring your forearms together down each side of their nose. Slowly but firmly apply gentle pressure down and outward, ironing out both sides of their face. This represents bringing them through the birth canal—ever so slowly, they are being born again.

Part Four: Rebirth

These moves complete the birthing process. Begin by saying, "Now, take the first breath to your new life." Instruct them to inhale deeply, and slide both your hands underneath their back, and prepare to slide your hands down toward their sacrum. You will need a fair amount of oil on your hands, arms, and the table underneath their back, to have enough glide for this move.

With the receiver inhaling, glide your hands down their back, one hand on either side of the spine, placing them just above the sacrum. Instruct them to exhale, "Now let it all go!" As they release the breath they have been holding, press your finger pads up into the channels along the spine on both side of the spine firmly, just above the sacrum. Then begin gliding very slowly up their back, fingers pads digging into the channels, dredging them out along the spine. Pull all the way up on each side of their spine and continue the stroke up the back of their neck, stretching and picking up their head from underneath and lifting it up toward the sky, as far as possible.

Ideally, this stroke happens on one long, slow exhale but if they need to take a second breath, that's fine. As they begin to inhale again ever so slowly, very gently place their head back on the table and allow them to relax in stillness.

Laulima: Laying On of Hands

Laulima, or the laying on of hands, is the finish to this ritual. Place your hands lightly with palms over the eye sockets or on the top of the head. Visualize a waterfall of aloha light coming down through the top of your head into your heart and out the palms of your hands onto their face. Take several deep breaths and just let the waterfall of aloha pour into them.

Soul Retrieval

When someone has been abused physically, emotionally, or sexually as a child, most often it was buried deep within their subconscious at the time it occurred. The body takes the trauma and stores it as a hurtful memory/image with a strong energetic charge attached, and locks it away to prevent any more pain. When these embedded memories of unprocessed feelings are triggered in a similar way, there can be a strong reaction as the memory rises to the surface to be expressed and finally healed. This is a delicate procedure involving witnessing, acknowledging and releasing. As the client goes into the memories and emotions, you must become the anchor for unconditional compassion, steadfast and fully present.

Preparation: The receiver lies on a bed or massage table faceup. They can wear light, loose clothing. If they like, they can use a sheet or light blanket to cover their body.

To begin: During any extreme trauma, part of the soul tends to leave the body when this happens. The result is a fragmentation of the soul, a compartmentalizing within the consciousness where part of the soul becomes walled off, and part of the person becomes trapped in the age they were when they were traumatized. Later in life, when triggered, this often shows up as an escape mechanism in response to intensity. All parts of the soul need to be reintegrated and brought together into present time.

A prayer is said to set the intention for release and reclamation. Encourage the client to call to mind a time when they were traumatized. Have them share their story and all the feelings associated with the trauma. When they have connected to the root of the trauma or memories in their mind and their body, ask the receiver to call back any lost parts of their soul that may have been detached and left somewhere when the incident occurred. Remember that the receiver's own breath is the greatest mover of their energy, the greatest transformer of their emotions and feelings. Conscious breathing along with sincere proclamations can turn a breakdown into a breakthrough and in its wake, return one to peace. During the process you can have them create movements and gestures to make this more real for them.

Now let's explore some simple ideas that can assist your healing work to release trauma and facilitate a soul retrieval.

Assist the client to stay present and grounded. We highly recommend you help them to voice what they are feeling so that they can stay connected in this process with you. As they speak, sincerely acknowledge them for what they are feeling and saying so they can feel heard. If anxiety or panic show up, help the client to stay present by getting them to breathe slowly and look around the room, to see that there's nothing to be afraid of. Slow conscious breathing is the key to staying calm when a traumatic or anxious vibration arises. Keep them grounded, touch the person, look in their eyes, and perhaps have them drink some water, to keep them in the present moment. Ask them to share what they are experiencing, holding them in grace as their story becomes unglued and their feelings begin to flow, discharging the emotional infection or toxicity.

Acknowledge the trauma and release its energetic charge. When a strong emotional charge is stored in the body such as jealousy, hate, grief, anger, resentment, or fear, the inner child needs a safe container to express these feelings. Ask the person to connect to the child within them and give it a voice, calling assistance from a higher power to transmute all the energetics associated with their memory. Guide them into acceptance of the story as just a story. Some clients may have to relive the memory. If they show signs of moving into a panic attack, their body may begin to shake, contort, or become rigid, as it begins to recall these hurtful memories. It is very important to stay extremely attentive to these waves for acceptance and healing as they arise to the surface. Show them how they are now safe in this present moment with you in a sacred healing temple. To release the negative charge in a healthy way, they must completely forgive the people involved (including themselves) and what took place.

You can open a dialog to reclaim everyone's innocence in their story, by allowing the person to share their memories and feelings. Show them how their story has been running their life and has caused them enough pain. I often use the metaphor of their story as just a scene in a movie replaying—it's not real. Ask them: "What lesson have you learned from this experience? How will you feel when the memory of this trauma no longer bothers you? What would that look like to you?" Offer them a vision of how free they will be without it. We often do a series of deep Ha breaths to process and "flush" the emotional charge.

Transmute the energy and reintegrate all parts of the soul. Once the hurtful memory has been discharged, envelop the client in a loving light with total compassion. Call for help from a higher power to transmute any energy associated with the events surrounding the issue. It is often helpful to recite along with them: *I'm sorry, please forgive me, thank you, I love you* to dispel any unclean energy that's ready to be released. After the forgiveness process is activated, assist the client to call all parts of their soul back to them by telling them to breathe deeply. As they breathe deeply, have them reach out and pull their soul back energetically. Have them make a gesture, opening their arms wide and hugging that part of their soul that's being retrieved, placing it in their body as they repeat the mantra. You can place your hands wherever you are guided on to their body—assisting to ground them.

Entity Removal

When there was extreme trauma in the family history, often the souls of the ancestors involved have so much unresolved that they do not ascend into the light—they remain earthbound. These earthbound spirits lack enough life-force energy to ascend, and they need help. It is our responsibility to assist these spirits to ascend, and this in turn assists the evolution of the entire family lineage. These spirits are seeking resolution and direction.

If the client has been abused, sometimes there is an energetic tie between them and their abuser. Because there is a hole created in the aura (or soul) of the person who was traumatized, this becomes an opening where a spirit can attach to the living person. Sometimes an ancestral spirit will attach itself to a descendant who is repeating a similar pattern. Other times it is just a dark mass of energy. Whatever the trauma, it begins a negative cycle of the person leaking their energy into these spirits or energetic forms that do not belong, creating imbalance in the body, mind, and spirit. 'Unihipili is the Hawaiian word for this lingering of unwanted, sticky attachments—"the soul that clings."

This can also involve patterns and events from past lives with energetic attachments to souls that were involved in traumatic events from other lifetimes. These can all be cleared and addressed over time, peeling back the layers like an onion.

"Conventional medical care ends at death, and this is a blessing for many who spend their last days in the hospital. On the other hand, shamans know that sometimes the soul is confused after death and cannot find its way to the next world without help. In fact, with sudden violent death or suicide, the departed person is often unaware of having left his or her body. The soul may wander about confounded by its inability to get what it wants. Coming across someone else whose defenses are weak, the dead may enter 'holes' or gaps in that person's soul. Once inside, the dead person manipulates the life of the live one. This is the most common form of possession."—Eliot Cowan, *Plant Spirit Medicine.*

This is a drain on the energy of the person and can cause all kinds of destructive behavior. This dysfunctional cycle can attract other energies that also stick in the body, creating depression, confusion, addictive tendencies, and fatal disease. The negative pattern lives on through the descendant until they are ready to raise their vibration and create a healthier pattern in their own life. It is essential for the soul's journey to realize one's true path and their true purpose in life, and to take steps toward aligning themselves with their divinity, facilitating new patterns that promote well-being. If the person heals the issues that created the hole in their soul, they can once again become a whole and integrated being, free of any other entities that may have been leaching off their energy.

Preparation: The receiver lies on a bed or massage table faceup. They can wear light, loose clothing. If they like, they can use a sheet or light blanket to cover their body. It is sometimes helpful to have the room dimly lit, with a candle burning on your altar and a smudge wand available to smudge the room, yourself, and the receiver. (See section on smudging for directions on the various techniques.)

To begin:

1. *Change the pattern, and raise the frequency*

   A prayer is said to set the intention for the liberation and release of the unwanted energies, inviting Jesus, the Holy Spirit, God, or ke Akua nui to assist. When the person who the soul is attaching to, begins to make choices based on love, rather than fear, the hole in their aura becomes healed, and the energetic ties connected to the earthbound spirit are loosened, weakened. The entity becomes disturbed because it is no longer being fed by the person's depression or despair. Sometimes it will try to reengage the person in negative behavior to keep its place in their body. If the person stays on track by not feeding the dysfunctional pattern, the unwanted spirit will have to leave because there's no way to remain attached. This "lost soul" can then be guided back into pure divine light once again. If the host engages in the behavior that attracts the negative energies, the spirit will remain attracted to them, and the pattern will continue until some form of intervention takes place. If this does not happen, the spirit may begin to hook itself back into that person or look for a new host, one that carries a similar pattern or issue that needs to be resolved.

2. *Order the entity to leave*

   To free themselves, the person coming to you for healing can consciously, lovingly and firmly order this "being" to leave their body and direct them into the light. This is the first part of an energetic soul retrieval. In some cases, it is not time for the spirit to leave yet because the person has not received the full lesson through the connection. In this case, you can still order the being to leave, expecting its imminent liberation, while allowing for more time for the detachment to take place. Have them speak to the energy first in their own words, and then have the person use the words "By the authority of my soul, I order you to leave my body now, and return to the light!" Have them take a deep breath and exhale out, releasing the energy.

3. *Call back your power*
   As a healer, you can participate in retrieving aspects of your receiver's soul that are attached to these unwarranted patterns, calling back their precious energy from leaking out through these attachments, and integrating the energy back into their energetic matrix.

   You can have the person use the words "I hereby reclaim all parts of my soul that have been lost, fragmented, or distorted because of this pattern. I call to all parts of me to come back, to come together now as one."

4. *Clear the energy, cut the cords*
   You can pull dark forms of energy out of their aura, and detach the energy connecting the entity to the client. An *oki* (cut) can be performed, which is a cutting

of the cord attached to the being that you are releasing. These parasitical beings draw energy from the energy field, causing all manner of distortion and leaving their host vulnerable and unbalanced. When the entity is released, there is a space left behind that needs to be filled. If there are rips or tears in your client's auric field, they must be repaired and sealed with sacred light after releasing the one that has been attached. Use intuitive hand movements with intention to clear the energy and smooth out any rough areas in the energetic field of the receiver. Have the receiver take several deep breaths, asking them to fill their aura with their own light. Smudging can be used here to clean and clear the aura as well as to protect the person and yourself.

5. *Call the angels to deliver the spirit to the light*
   We often find that in a very deep lomi healing, spirits are easily liberated and brought into the light. They are most often eager to be set free, and they just need to be acknowledged, loved, and given a definitive direction. Once they are shown the path to the light, they will cooperate and move on. There is much help from the upper realms available to assist these lost souls on their journey into the light. There are angels who have been assigned the role of ushering lost souls into the light. When you call to them, the guardian angels gather above the table and open a portal from above (which has often been described as a spiraling

funnel of light). The angels and spirit helpers take the earthbound spirit and lovingly pull it upward into the upper realms. It is a very beautiful process, nothing to be feared. Sometimes several beings all decide to leave at the same time, as though they have been waiting for an opportunity to move into the next level of their evolution, and are happy to go toward the light. When you feel an attached entity or a being that needs to be moved into the light, it is often helpful for you and/or the client to use the words "I set you free!" Then direct the energy upward, breathing it into the portal. Every being is simply seeking to be loved into the light.

Occasionally, you may encounter more challenging or serious cases of possession that you cannot handle. Just as before, this is nothing to be feared. In cases of challenging possession, surround yourself in a protective light, trust that love prevails all trauma, be patient, and know that the matter can be resolved in time. Be attentive and check in with the receiver to see how they are feeling. Keep doing all the methods we mentioned until you feel complete. Continue to pray for the receiver—let go and let God! When you feel complete, finish by praying in gratitude.

The Golden Cocoon Activation

When a healing session is complete, this delicate moment often requires sacred ritual to implant a permanent impression of alteration within the receiver, affirming on all levels of their being that a change has taken place. With this in mind, Kealohi created the golden cocoon as a celestial rite of passage, a process that encapsulates the healing, sealing it in cosmic golden light. It can be used as a finish to a Kahi Loa session or at the end of a massage, or just on its own as a light body activation where the receiver can receive healing, messages, or visions from spirit.

Components of the Activation Process

+ *Part one:* Casting of stars

+ *Part two:* Building the golden cocoon

  » Inhaling sparks of sacred light while slowly pulling the sheet

  » Filling all the cells of the bones, the blood, and the flesh (especially the organs) with light

  » Filling the entire aura with sacred golden sparks of pure white-light

  » Balancing neurological circuits while angels weave the golden cocoon

+ *Part three:* Activating the golden cocoon

  » Calling in kanaka—a human spirit

  » Kaulike—the touch of an angel—final activation of the cocoon

  » Rainbow sweeps—acknowledging the blessings of heaven and earth

The first part is called the "casting of stars," invoking a connection to the heavens. The second part we call the "golden cocoon" because it creates, activates, and seals the receiver in a potent field of golden-white light within and around their body.

In the third part, the client calls a being who is or has been human (living and passed away are both fine) whom they would like to be blessed by to further accentuate a healing connection of their choosing. In this final stage of the activation, the healing is done by spirit and continues as they lie on the table in their cocoon, morphing into the newest, highest version of themselves.

Many clients have stated that during this portion of the session they felt the spirit of the one they chose touching them or actually speaking to them telepathically. One woman had chosen her father who had passed away several years before, and after this process, tears were flowing down her cheeks. As she did not share with me who she had chosen, I saw her tears and asked if she was all right. She said yes and then asked me if she could be alone with her father for just a while longer because he was in the room, holding her hand.

The Casting of Stars

The casting of stars is used to symbolize the larger, outer sense of who we are as a cosmic being. Abraham, Serge, Harry, Sherman, and many other great teachers have made us aware that we are one with the entire universe. We each have access to the entire cosmos from within. To empower this idea, a reconnecting from soul to stars gesture was developed using a sheet to create a dramatic beginning to the ritual. This process involves calling to our star ancestors, breathing in the mana from the stars, and blowing it into the sheet. Then like a magician might do, the sheet is thrown over the receiver, covering them with a blanket of stars.

Preparation: The receiver lies on a bed or massage table faceup. They can wear light, loose clothing. Cover their body with a sheet. (If used as a closing to a massage session, the receiver can be unclothed but may need a smaller drape tucked around the breasts and pelvic area.)

To begin: Pick up the sheet, holding its length horizontal. Hands should be a little more than shoulder-width apart; stand on one side of the table. Raise your arms outstretched above your head high in front of you between you and the massage table. Now look up. Set your intention and call in the blessing of the star ancestors. Breathe in the energy of the stars, visualizing the Milky Way and all the constellations above you coming into your lungs, as you inhale through your mouth. And then, blow into the sheet, filling the sheet with stars as you exhale fully.

Bring the sheet down a little so your arms are outstretched in front of you while holding the sheet quite firmly. Snap the sheet three times by bringing your hands a little closer together and pulling them apart quickly. Now cast the sheet full of stars: throw it over the person as if you are casting a net to catch fish, horizontally about two or three feet above the receiver's body. Allow it to float down, covering them completely, enveloping them in a blanket of stars from their cosmic brothers and sisters of light from all known and unknown universes.

The Golden Cocoon

Preparation: Turn the lights in the room down low. The receiver should be facing up, covered with a sheet up to their neck and down over their toes. In most cases, your receiver will be in a very deep trance as their healing session comes to a close. If the receiver is unclothed, be sure to have another drapery secured in place over the groin, and another secured over the breast area if needed for privacy, because you will be removing the top sheet.

To begin: Instruct your receiver by saying: "Imagine that the room is filled with sparks of golden light, coming down from the cosmos. These tiny sparks of light are swirling and spinning in every direction, and they are magnetized by your love. I want you now to begin a breathing pattern. Breathe in these little, tiny golden sparks of white light. Inhale them deeply into the cells of your body, beginning at the tips of your toes. Breathe in these sparks and fill every single cell in your feet with these tiny sparks, overflowing each cell with this loving gift of cosmic light."

As they begin to breathe in stardust, stand above their head and very slowly take the edges of the sheet at their shoulders, and pull the sheet up over their body *very*, very slowly to uncover the feet, then the ankles, shins, knees, hips, hands and belly, elbows, shoulders, neck, and face. While you are pulling the sheet, guide them through each part of the body as it is exposed. Instruct them to fill each and every cell of the parts of the body the bottom of the sheet uncovers.

Repeat the following over and over as you drag the sheet up the body. "Breathe deeply, and fill every single cell of your body with these exquisite particles of pure divine light. Filling the bones, the blood, and the flesh—filling and overflowing each cell with tiny sparks of golden, white light. Filling, filling, filling every single cell with this precious gift of cosmic light!" (Because you have secured your smaller drapery over the groin and/or breast area, you can pull the sheet all the way up and off the face; this way every part receives the blessing of this electric, holy light generated from their spirit, and their 'aumakua, through the power of their imagination.)

Filling the Aura with Light

After the sheet has been fully removed, walk around to the side of the table and perform the casting of stars once more, covering them in a blanket of stars from the Milky Way. Once the sheet has been cast again and is flat on top of them, tuck it neatly under their chin and instruct them, saying: "Now begin to breathe once again, filling your aura with electric golden sparks of light. And as you exhale, please breathe these beautiful particles of light out into your aura, filling your aura with golden white light. Now take a few more breaths, and as you exhale, expand your aura out into the whole room, filling the room with tiny stars, just like the Milky Way!"

Balancing Neurological Circuits
While Weaving the Golden Cocoon

You will now begin to weave their energetic cocoon. Hold each set of points for at least seven seconds while intentionally connecting the energy between the points. While you do this, your receiver has been participating by filling their aura with little stars of golden light. Stand at the side of the table next to your receiver's right hand.

1. Locate the upper right corner (the corner closest to you) of their pubic bone, with your right middle finger. Plant the tip of your finger firmly on the top corner.

2. Now locate a point on their eyebrow closest to you near the center of their face, on the upper inside ridge of the eye socket. Firmly plant your left middle finger there. Imagine the energy connecting between these two points while softly humming, toning, or repeating, "I am, I am, I am …" over and over, activating an energetic connection between these points.

3. Next, cross over to their left eyebrow point with your left middle finger while keeping your right finger on the right corner of the pubic bone, again intoning "I am" repeatedly, running energy back and forth with your intention. The connection is now diagonal, running from the person's left eyebrow and right corner of the pubic bone.

4. Now move your right middle finger across to the other upper left corner of their pubic bone. Both of your fingers are now on the person's left side, pubic bone, and brow points. Hum, intone, or softly repeat "I am," running the energy.

5. Next, bring your left middle finger back to the person's right eyebrow point. Visualize a diagonal arc of energy, mumbling "I am" repeatedly, running back and forth with your eyes. There are four polarity points which have been balanced so far.

It's time to call to the angels to gather above the table. Ask the angels to take the golden white sparks of light and begin spinning a golden cocoon around their aura. Tell the receiver, "Now it is time for us to invite all the angels and ancestors here to weave this light into a golden cocoon of loving and healing protection; spiraling ribbons of golden light all around your body. Around and around they go, from your head to your toes, spinning and weaving a beautiful golden cocoon around your body.

6. While they focus on this, move your right middle finger to the middle of their pubic bone, on the top ridge.

7. Place your left middle finger to a point just under their nose and above their upper lip, in the philtrum (divot). Visualize energy running from their tailbone up the back of their spine, over their head to your other finger.

8. Finally, move your left middle finger centered just below their lower lip and run the energy from the pubic ridge up the front of the body to under their lips. Now you have completed balancing their nervous system and can activate the golden cocoon.

Kaulike: Spirit-Assisted Activation

Upon completing the polarity-balancing-series for the nervous system, we begin the activation; incubating the newest, highest version of their soul's journey here on Earth. We continue with a technique learned from Dr. King called kaulike, or "to balance evenly." This is also the final module we use in a Kahi Loa healing session called kanaka, used to call to the human kingdom. This process involves connecting with a spirit that has been, or is still human. Some people will pick one of their parents or children, a partner, or a loved one who is alive or who has passed on. Some choose Jesus, Mary, Archangel Michael, or a spirit guide they would like to become more familiar with.

The Touch of an Angel

Engage the receiver by saying, "To finally activate your golden cocoon, I would like you to choose a divine being to be touched by. This can be someone still in a body, or someone who has been in a body. You can call to this being silently or out loud; open to your heart to receive all their healing blessings. When you are holding this being firmly in your heart, nod your head and I will touch you as their presence."

When the receiver signals they are ready by nodding their head, raise and open your arms outstretched to receive the blessing of the spirit they chose to be with. After merging with the spirit, bring your hands to your heart, allowing that spirit's love for the one on the table to come through you to bless the receiver.

Connecting the Chakras

Preparation: This is a light touch, yet very intentional contact using a few fingerpads on each of the chakras at first, then connecting with the major joints. Both series of points begin at the head and move down the body. First you leapfrog your hands down the chakra points, so that there is always contact with one hand while the other hand is moving to a new chakra. As you touch each place on their body, hold the thought and the feeling of "I love you. I love you. I love you," allowing the blessing of the spirit to flow through you.

To begin: After the receiver nods their head indicating they are ready for the activation, stand on one side of the massage table, place a few finger-pads from one hand on their crown chakra (the top of their head) and a few fingerpads from the other hand on their brow chakra, (the forehead). Hold the first two points, crown and brow, long enough to give time for the human spirit they picked to plug in to them fully before moving your finger that was on the top of the head to the throat chakra, connecting the third eye to the throat chakra.

Move the hand that was touching the forehead and place it on the heart, connecting the throat and heart. Hold for about seven seconds. Take the hand that was touching the throat to the top of the belly just below the sternum, connecting the heart to the solar plexus. Hold these points for about seven seconds, then take the hand that was touching the heart and place it just over the navel (sacral chakra). Connect the energy between the two points while silently repeating "I love you," touching them as the spirit of the one they have chosen.

Anuenue: The Rainbow
Connecting Heaven and Earth

When you reach the person's navel center as you are going down the body, place one open palm (fingers together) three inches over the crown of their head and the other open palm three inches below their root chakra, at the base of the spine, *not* touching the body. Sending love through your hands, visualize a rainbow with one end at the bottom of the tailbone and one end over their crown.

Move your hands up slowly into an arc closer together, connecting both hands over their heart about two feet above their body. Send the rainbow into their heart. This gesture bathes the crown and the root chakras in rainbow light and unites in their heart.

Connecting the Joints

The second part of kaulike brings the "touch of an angel" to balance all the major joints in the body. Instead of leapfrogging, you hold left and right sides of the body and move both at the same time. Place a few fingerpads from each hand very gently on each side of their body at the joints, beginning at the sides of the jaw, then shoulders, elbows, wrists, hips, knees, ankles, and toes. Work your way down the body, finishing at the big toe. Hold each set of points for three or four seconds.

Anuenue: Earth to Earth Rainbow, Acknowledging the Body

Seal the session with a sweeping gesture, beginning on the ground just beneath their feet, at the end of the table. Root the rainbow into the earth, bringing a blessing from the earth. Lift it up with your arms outstretched, sweeping up from over their feet, their legs, over their upper body, their head, and back down to the floor, offering the blessing back to the earth.

This completes the acknowledgment of their existence as a human, made of flesh and bone. Our body comes from the earth and one day it will return to the earth. Give thanks.

Anuenue: Heaven to Heaven Rainbow, Acknowledging the Spirit

To acknowledge their existence as spirit, stand at the head of the table (the end just above their head) and face the receiver. Reach your arms high, outstretched above their head, palms up, open wide to the gift of aloha light that's being offered to them from spirit. Visualize receiving a golden sphere of light in your open hands. Upon receiving it, pull the energy down from above and share it with the person on the table. Bring the blessing from above their head, sweeping your arms all the way across the top of their body, from over their head and chest, down over their legs and toes, and back up to heaven. This acknowledges the spirit that dwells within them, as them and for them. Our spirit is formed from light and someday will return to light.

Into *Po*—Cover the Eyes

Gently place an eye pillow or folded pillowcase over the person's eyes. The angels will take over at this point; you get to rest and witness, holding sacred space for the miracle to root more deeply into their being. We have often felt the room fill up with beings at this point while praying in gratitude for them. This is another opportunity for the person's ancestors to also be present, touching them in their own loving way. Sit in a chair or lie down on the floor next to the massage table and merge with their bliss, present within and around them, flooding the temple space with heaven's impeccable presence. While the person rests, incubating inside their cocoon, the perfect selection of soft music will further enhance the depth of the experience. This is a joyous moment, floating in a timeless sea of infinite potential, the cosmic realm of the kahuna and all ascended beings.

A strong beginning and a strong ending is imperative for any ritual to be effective. By beginning with the opening protocols outlined in this book, performing some shamanic bodywork techniques on the back and front of the body, and then finally ending here, creating a field of highly charged healing energy that spirit can work through, your receiver will have a shamanic experience that they will remember forever on some level. Perhaps they will commune with an ancestor who has a direct message for them, or perhaps they will journey very deep into their cocoon, and then emerge with renewed innocence. The possibilities are infinite. Enjoy this experience!

12

We Are Never Alone

'Ike aku, 'ike mai, kokua aku, kokua
mai; pela iho la ka nohana 'ohana.
Recognize and be recognized, help
and be helped; such is family life.

If you have made it to this point in the book, you likely have some ideas and inspiration of how to use sacred shamanic bodywork and Hawaiian healing principles to transform your life and the lives of others. Perhaps you would like to begin to experiment and practice some of these ideas but do not have access to a teacher. We would like to encourage you to harness the assistance of the helpful beings in the spirit world who play a very important role in everyone's healing journey. In truth, we are never truly alone—a myriad of spirit guides will come to us when called upon with an open, humble heart, holding positive expectations. This is the essence of faith, and with time our connection becomes even more effective. It is up to us, to the best of our ability, to believe in a higher power and open to receive the guidance. Our ancestors and spirit guides do not judge us. From their perspective, they can only love us—because only love is real. In this regard, they can be called upon for their wisdom, and we can put our trust in our guides to assist us in developing our healing skills, energizing our hands when we touch someone.

Seeing Energy and Communicating with Spirit Guides

Whether you are aware of it or not, there are many beings watching over us all the time. We cannot always see them because they live in a different dimension or frequency than we do.

Human beings have been gifted with great power to connect with and access our ancestors and our personal guardian angels, spirit guides, ascended masters, and many other beings to whom we may be drawn. Though it may seem imagined or created by the mind, it may carry a very strong significance on an emotional level. On a spiritual level, it may influence you by opening the way for cocreating a miracle. With patience and practice, one can begin to hear the voices of their guides, and channel pertinent messages from the spirit realm. You can learn to communicate with these beings, and watch what happens when you believe; they are really here to assist you in your evolution.

Open yourself to the possibility that more is going on than we may be able to see with the naked eye. Imagine that you could train your eyes to see in a whole new way, revealing what has been hidden from your vision all this time. It has been recorded in history that when the very first explorers from Europe began to visit remote island locations, the islanders would look out over the ocean, and many of them could not see the ships of the explorers, because they had no mental concept or reference for ships in their perception of reality. They had no ability to see something that they did not know existed, so their visual world didn't extend that far. It wasn't until someone who was trained to see beyond the normal realm of vision could sense something. Perhaps the shaman of the tribe looked out over the water and adjusted or shifted his perception so that the ships appeared in the distance, right before his very eyes. Just as these people in ancient times had to learn how to see the ships, it is not possible for us to see various realms of spirit, until we adjust our perception to be able to see in this way.

EXERCISE: Seeing and Feeling Energy

To Prepare: Sit comfortably in a quiet room or outside in nature.

To begin: To practice shifting your perception or see energy, squint your eyes and let things go a little out of focus, bringing into view the energy that surrounds all things. You can do this by sitting and looking at your two hands, holding them about two feet from your face. Move them toward each other a little, feeling the energy coming between your hands, and gazing into the space where the fingers connect to the space around them. Or you can lie down and gaze up at a tree, looking at the space where the branches connect to the sky. Close your eyes, and then slowly open them. Then slowly close them again and open them slowly again. After a while, focusing and unfocusing your gaze, you may begin to see energy coming off your fingers, or feel a tingling or warm energy in your hands. If you practice this out in nature, you will begin to see energetic exchanges taking place; what you focus/unfocus on will begin to glow. The Magic Eye-type books are really great for this kind of practice. By relaxing your eyes, and softening your gaze—not allowing what you think you should be seeing any attention—then what was hidden from your view before, will become visible and reveal a much wider spectrum of reality to you.

Developing a Navigational System of Omens and Signs

Each of us has a unique way to interpret the energy that weaves through us, as us, and for us, connecting us with all beings. For some, the spirit realm is felt more than seen. The presence of a spirit might send a physical sensation such as goosebumps, warmth, or the feeling of someone touching us. Look and listen for signs and omens, because active spirits can cause elemental energy in nature to animate, announcing their presence to get our attention. They're offering to communicate something of value to us, conveying some helpful information that will open us to see or feel things differently. There are messengers all around us, all the time, if we are paying attention.

When the unseen wants you to pay attention, there are many signs that usually go un-noticed, that become unblocked, when we tune into the present moment, fully aware, deeply listening. Ask the helpful spirits to give you a sign when they are wanting to inform you. Then trust and open to your own intuition to read the signs that come.

You can associate different animals or birds with different meanings, and spirit will send the animal or a picture of that animal to tell you if you are on the right track or not. Be sure to note if the animal is dead or alive, its state of health, its behavior, and what you were thinking when it appeared.

Angels seem to enjoy communication through light and sound. On the balcony at home, we have often heard the unseen ones hit only one note on the wind chime, ringing slowly four times to get our attention while the other wind chime (several feet away) isn't moving because there is no wind, at all. They may knock an object off a shelf or make a door open or close. You may be sitting in your living room and the lights start to flicker. Or you may be walking down the road and suddenly the light changes somehow, a streetlight goes on or off, or the clouds arrange themselves in a very peculiar way. Notice what you were thinking or talking about when the mysterious change in your environment happened.

These signs are always noticeable when we can relax into our unity with all that is. You see, because they are not physical beings, they will gently offer their assistance, but they will be subtle in their approach; their "will" is not imposed on us. They cannot influence our physical dimension unless we invite or call them here, through our will. If you are wanting a deeper connection to a spirit guide, greet them, acknowledge them with gratitude, and welcome them into your heart and your space of existence. Then open wide to receive any sublime messages. Your guides will begin to make themselves known in their own unique way. Just pay attention and trust whatever comes to you as you move through your day.

Through a reverent acknowledgment, you can feel the ancestors and spirit beings all around you. Their love is palpable. They want you to know that they are willing to assist you in any way they are able, to promote your well-being and the well-being of your loved ones. Ask them for help on specific issues in your life. If you are wanting assistance with healing yourself, they can work with your ancestors to guide you to the right teachers and the right experiences to provide you with your needs at the time. Perhaps they guided you to pick up this book. Here's the most interesting part of all this. As we call them into this plane of existence through song, chant, and prayer, to assist us in our healing work, we actually become guided in our service to them, as grace enters into our life in greater and greater ways.

As we grow in awareness through experience, we see that our experience here on earth is temporary. That beyond our body, we have an identity, an essence, a spirit made of light that lives on forever. The guardians and guides serve to remind us that there is more to life than meets the eye, and more power available to us than we can imagine.

13

Nalu Pule O'o (Powerful Prayer Meditations)

Pule o'o (powerful prayer) creates *lokahi* (unity),
within an upward spiral for regenerating pono
(goodness), allowing divine-right-order to appear.
—Kealohi

Prayer is an act of devotion, a holy communion with our personal divinity. This means to connect deeply with the infinite power source of all life—the grace that resides within all beings and animates all things. No matter where we find ourselves or what's going on with our lives, we are one with all of creation. It's most effective to pray from this place of oneness with the source. For in this place, there is no lack, limit, or separation. Pray knowing that the prayer has already been answered. Careful listening during and after the prayer brings you guidance and comfort and helps to cultivate the courage that you need to mature, growing spiritually through all the circumstances you find yourself in. Learn to pray in gratitude all the time, and your life will become a river of love and blessings in action for all beings.

Prayer as Medicine

People come with all manner of brokenness, stuck emotions, and pain looking for relief or a way out of their circumstances. Many people think they are alone in their pain, helpless and victimized. When you sit down to pray with someone in need of a boost, you can shift their awareness to an inner strength and a profound faith that has access to the universal life source to resolve any earthly problem or challenge. All problems appear within an experience of separation from one's higher self (sometimes called the Godself). A prayer is a call for love to adjust our perspective of a situation. A deep prayer—one you can feel in your body— is a meditation, and when combined with conscious breathing, becomes medication. It can assist in shifting our viewpoint and our choices into a more manageable arrangement for all. A powerful prayer generates a positive trance state, to be applied when any situation requires an uplifting vibration. When you have a headache, you reach for medicine; when you feel fear and separation, you reach for prayer. A good prayer meditation is rooted in the highest underlying truth: **only love is real** and **God is all there is.** Everything else is an illusion or a misperception. When you design your prayer around this fundamental truth, you begin to see that everything is sacred. Everything connects to a divine design, and the prayer is a way to attune yourself to this divine current of energy that exists for us to employ and enjoy. Everything that does not serve you falls away, and you can move forward in the right direction from a place of trust, renewed strength, and clarity.

Praying for Others

You can use prayer to assist others with long-distance healing. This is done by connecting with the highest frequency in and around you, attuning yourself to it, and then sending it to the soul of another, through the "spirit channel." You can draw upon divine light and grace, through blessing and acknowledgment, at the beginning or end of each day and send this aloha nui through the "inner-net" to anyone who needs healing. The higher self of the receiver is always receptive to loving blessings. You can pray for the health and well-being of another as long as you have no agenda to interfere with their life path or their free will. Pray that your receiver will remember their true identity as love. Through sacred vision, see them as perfect, whole, innocent, and free. Summon their guardian angels to shine light on them, to assist them to find it in their heart to forgive, release, and let go of "cherished wounds," and any unforgiveness and expired agreements. Pray that their Divinity comes forward to bless their inner child so that they will be able to see their own innocence and the innocence of the ones who have played a part in hurting them or perhaps leaving them.

In praying for the healing of another, pray with gratitude that their soul cluster—their body, mind, and spirit that is their unique signature in this life—will realign in harmony and grace. If they share a story with you that is part of their healing, give the story to divinity and ask that you will be able to compassionately disengage from their story while listening carefully and receiving it into the Holy space you harbor for them. Pray for them to remember love because you know in your heart of hearts that only through our loving without conditions are we able to transcend all things. The presence of love creates a form of gravity for our soul that restores wholeness to our existence.

> *May the long time sun shine upon you,*
> *all love surround you,*
> *and the pure light within you*
> *guide your way on*
> —an Irish blessing

Prayer for Ho'oponopono

Prayer can lift what may feel like the heaviest burdens (stones) of fear and suffering, personal loss, guilt, anger, trauma, betrayal, and abandonment from your bowl of light. Lifting these hurtful issues as well as daily stresses and tensions is always a healthy practice for anyone, not just a shaman or healer. A good forgiveness prayer can and will relieve you from many heavy and uncomfortable circumstances that you may find yourself engaged in either personally or with others because it facilitates a definitive shift in perception to a higher level to lighten your load.

As Glenda Green says in her book *Love Without End: Jesus Speaks:*

To solve a problem it is first necessary to view it from a higher level, thus gaining a larger perspective. In the areas of physical healing this is obvious. A physician or a medical facility can only arrest an illness, keep it from progressing, reduce infection, and provide conditions where healing may occur. The actuality of healing is always a miracle that happens on a higher level through the restoration of wholeness. No matter what the problem, healing always comes from a higher level.

In ancient times in Hawaii, traditional ho'oponopono was practiced every night with the whole family before bed. The stories tell us that all generations were present in the family room for this to happen. This was done to clear any resentments anyone may be carrying so as not to take those resentments into their dreamtime. In this way, they would sleep with a clear conscience and wake refreshed, renewed, and without hindrance from any grievances from the previous day. It is still a good practice today, never go to bed angry.

It is good practice to clear your conscience every night when you lay your head on the pillow. Similar to a bedtime prayer, you are honoring sacred innocence within yourself and others, making use of gratitude within forgiveness.

The following prayer created by Morrnah Simeona is for personal healing. It is used for clearing your body and releasing the inner child of any negative ideas, thoughts, or beliefs your mind has clung to over the years. It uses the mind to focus by taking the hand of the child and guiding it to open up to the higher self and receive clarity and guidance. By clearing these attachments from the body-mind, you are removing rocks from your bowl of light, opening a clear space for higher guidance, inspiration, and beliefs that will bring healing energies into our whole lifestream. You can recite this prayer to bring pono to your soul cluster from your mental self (mother) to your physical self (child) with help from your higher self or 'aumakua (father). Appeal to the inner child that lives within your body to let go of all the negative things you have been telling it and feeding it.

Divine Creator, Father, Mother, Child as One.

*Oh my child, will you forgive me for all my errors,
in thoughts, words, deeds, and actions I have
accumulated and subjected you to over time?*

As your Mother today,

*I forgive you for all your fears, resentments, insecurities,
guilts and frustrations.*

*Come and hold my hand, and reverently, ask the Father,
our 'aumakua, to join us and hold our hands.*

*As a unit of two, please ask the Father to join us and make
the three of us a unit of one. Let love flow from me to you
and from us to the Father.*

Let the Divine Creator embrace us in the Divine Circle of love.

In repeating this prayer, focus your energy upon resolving the *pilikia* (trouble) by clearing the subconscious until the problem has lifted. Call on your higher self to undo the negative projections by repeating: "I'm sorry, please forgive me, thank you, I love you."

For Peaceful Sleep

Heal your body to sleep by filling your body with light and love. Close your eyes and breathe deeply, inhaling light into every body part, beginning with your feet. Use "I love you" as your mantra. Imagine pure light is filling all the cells of your toes, then your ankles. Move up your legs to your knees, breathing light into all your bones, into your upper legs, relaxing your hips, and your whole upper torso, breathing light into your belly, your liver, your stomach, your open chest, and all around your radiant heart! Breathe and feel the light that is glowing from your heart and traveling through the blood to all your body parts. Breathe the light from your heart out your arms now, all the way to the tip of each finger, one at a time. Bathe in this glow and be at peace with your day as you lay it down to rest along with your body-mind. Say these words:

I praise this day, I forgive this day. I release this day, I bless this day.

Thank you, God for this day.

Thank you for all the love that was shared, in every moment, with everyone.

May all beings rest in peace this night.

I love you, and I'm grateful to be one with you and all creation!

Mana Meditation

Close your eyes and begin a deep breathing pattern. Place your tongue on the roof of your mouth and keep it there for this practice. Breathe light in through your crown at the top of your head, drawing it into your heart area. On the exhale, fill your belly with light. Focus on inhaling abundant, pure, light-filled love, in through the top of your head. As you exhale slowly, deposit it in your belly. Soon you will feel a glowing warmth there. Do this until you feel peace within. To enhance this meditation, place your hands on your belly.

From Dreaming to Streaming

So many dreams will never come true; it's often the ones you could never plan that actually do. Playing in the waves of time and space, we nourish each other, revealing our belonging.

The sun blazes down as the mother wakes. She hears children playing at heaven's gate. Glowing warmth opens the heart, take a deep breath and let the light shine, total surrender to the current of love divine, rippling and healing everything in its path! "Now" is our guide, "where" is always here; this "moment" is all we are—pure awareness—as love.

Have no fear, love is here. No longer dreaming, we're now streaming—blissful radiance.

Prayer to Open the Heart

Say this prayer with love as you breathe in and out, expanding through your heart chakra.

- *Pu'u wai hamama* (My heart is open)

- Divine creator, father, mother, child as one,

- I open my heart to receive all your blessings:
  Pu'u wai hamama...

- I open my heart to reveal who I am as you:
  Pu'u wai hamama...

- I open my heart to share these sacred gifts with all:
  Pu'u wai hamama...

- I open my heart to the blessing of a life filled with purpose: *Amama*: Amen—so it is!

- *E aloha pau ole*: Love has no end

To Open a Healing Session

As a facilitator, you can work with the person receiving healing to form and recite with devotion, an opening blessing/prayer to start the session. Have the receiver set one clear intention for what they would like to release during their session and one clear intention for what they would like to call into their life and speak it into the prayer. This protocol sets the foundation of a definitive healing tone for the session.

Here is an example of a prayer we often use:

'Aumakua, Aloha, Mahalo! (Guardian spirits, we love you, we thank you!)

I call to all our guardians, guides, and ancestors for support in this healing.

I call for our divine higher selves, the greatness of spirit to come forward and bless the divine child within each of us.

I call to Great Spirit to bring forth the perfect wave of aloha to bring healing nourishment and bless … (name the receiver) with divine love, to help them to release (insert their intentions here) … and bring them … (insert their intentions here).

To finish the prayer with a Hawaiian chant or blessing, here is a short blessing *pule* in Hawaiian created by Serge Kahili King that can be used in any ceremony or healing.

'Aumakua, mai ka po wai ola, ho ike a, mai ike ola. (Higher self, ancestors, bring forth the waters of life from heaven and manifest this blessing.)

Amama, ua noa, lele walea ku ala! (So Be it! This prayer is released. Fly off and manifest!)

A Healer's Proclamation to Ke Akua (Creator)

It takes courage to step out in the world and offer your healing energy to others. It helps to begin each day by offering yourself to be an instrument of healing, and trust that spirit will guide you every step of the way! This prayer opens the way for God to bring miracles of service into your life. You can say this when you are asked to take a big risk in helping someone heal and you want to establish a deeper flow within the abundant current of divine will and power.

Aloha ke Akua! (Loving greetings to the Creator)

We come thanking you for the gift of life today,
and for this opportunity to become closer to you,
through the loving service we give to others.

We can do this, because we are working for you,
God—the spirit of unity, harmony, and peace!

The Holy Spirit is always protecting us and watching over us.

This is God's work, and we are always safe to open and heal.

The greatest love and devotion will
always bring us the perfect people,
to create the perfect change,
at the perfect moment,
in the perfect manner,
in the perfect measure.
for a perfect shift to take place.

Amama, so be it! And so it is!

Mahalo nui ke Akua'

The Four Declarations of the Halau

You can become kahuna "waves of aloha" on someone's shore, sharing the blessing of well-being and gratitude with all who are invited into your healing temple. Yet before offering assistance to anyone else, it is wise to center yourself in meditation and/or prayer. You may use any prayer that works for you for harmonizing your soul cluster (or meditate in silence), making you a fountain of aloha and then offering this to others.

Here are the four declarations of the halau from Uncle Harry Jim's *Haumana Class Workbook*. They are designed for the lomi giver to recite before performing any healing. When spoken as a prayer for the purpose of activation, these declarations are powerful energetic tools that animate divinity into form, allowing heaven to show up on earth for you and your receiver.

1. My presence in the halau is a sacred manifestation from me to myself to shower gratitude, growth, and bliss to my whole being—and through me to the receiver.

2. I focus to enter and sustain my temple for lomilomi in the pu'u wai, the sacred space of the heart. From the heart and through the heart, the essence of my light, my 'uhane, supports, guides, and graces my touch.

3. I commit the energy of certainty to the abundance and perfection of my intuition as I am radiant in the light of aloha.

4. I will my will to compassionate disengagement, I am sustained by aloha, the breath of God is in our presence.

It is very important to fully understand the potency of these declarations. In the first, you are announcing that this space is created by you and for you to enjoy the healing process that is about to unfold. When you embody the feeling of gratitude, growth, and bliss, the receiver will pick up on this vibration and will begin to feel better while opening to their own divine nature.

In the second declaration, you are opening the portal of your sacred heart so that the greatness of your spirit can assist and support the bodywork you are doing.

In the third, you anchor yourself in the energy of certainty. You can trust your intuition and trust that you will do the perfect thing at the perfect time with perfect love.

In the fourth declaration, you are affirming that through compassionate disengagement, your will actually allows the healing to be done by the person on the table in cooperation with all the spirit guides: You do not use your own energy; you let the energy flow through you. You do not need to make anything happen; you just show up fully present with a willing heart to be present as a witness to the healing taking place with love. When we come from a place of compassionate disengagement, we do not take on any negative energy from the healing session, because the high vibration generated within the spirit of aloha transmutes all lower frequencies into pure light.

In reciting these declarations, you have given the healing work over to the energy of the halau, in trust that a miracle or shift in perception will take place. For a more in-depth understanding of Uncle Harry Jim's work, we highly recommend reading his book *Wise Secrets of Aloha*.

Prayer to Open to Christ Consciousness

Christ consciousness is the same type of frequency as aloha. It consists of pure unconditional love that is connected to a source of strength and guidance. Here's a powerful attunement prayer from Jesus, written in *The Way of Mastery*, published by the Shanti Christo Foundation:

> *May Christ alone dwell within and as this creation that I thought was myself.*
>
> *May Christ alone inform each thought, each breath, and each choice.*
>
> *May love direct each step.*
>
> *May love transform this journey through time, that in time I might truly know the reality of eternity, the sanctity of peace, the holiness of intimacy, and the joy of the Father's love.*
>
> *Amen*

Healing Prayer Meditations

When you offer prayer as medicine, so much unwanted energy can be cleared in what feels like no time because authentic prayer happens out-of-time. Ancient Hawaiians understood the power of the spoken word. Words were chosen carefully and spoken with intention and vibration, matching each word with emotion to give them more mana. So enjoy this process!

Here's the delicate process we share for activating the will to heal, committing to let go of judgments, to trust and surrender all misalignment to a higher power. You can use it on yourself, and offer it to others. Bring your passion into the words you are speaking. If you like, you can design your own variations of this prayer to be even more personal. Use whatever words you feel as most suitable, comfortable, and appropriate. If you don't resonate with saying "Holy Spirit" in the prayer, you can use "I trust and surrender to my highest good," "my own light," or "the light of my soul." Remember that the best results are attained by slow repetition with devotion. It can be done several times a day, during times of crisis, or we highly recommend that you recite this prayer/meditation before going to sleep at night, when the conscious mind has surrendered. When we sleep, there can be no resistance from that part of our mind that doesn't believe in miracles. This attunes you to self-healing and commits the body to letting go.

We suggest reciting this prayer for seven days before a bodywork session. Many clients have stated that they loved doing this prayer, as it helped them so much to align with their will to heal that when they finally arrived for their bodywork session, many things were easily released. Here's the format for using this as a protocol ritual.

Find a quiet and relaxing place to sit. Close your eyes and begin breathing deeply into your heart from your crown until you feel centered and ready to start. When you feel present and centered in your heart, open your eyes and read aloud the self-healing prayer—slowly with sincerity. When you are finished reading it, close your eyes and breathe it deeply into your whole body. Open your eyes and read it again. Slower this time. After the second time, close your eyes again and breathe this proclamation into all the cells of your body.

Open your eyes and read it a third time, taking a s-l-o-w deep breath in between each line, one line at a time.

Each time you repeat the prayer, say it slower and slower with more conviction, tasting each word and its potent ability to heal all misperceptions.

Repeat the entire prayer out loud at least three times or more, until you feel a substantial shift in your energy field as you drop deeper into it each time. You will feel it in your soul cluster when it's been fully activated. When you feel at one with your higher self, abide in silence, eyes closed, meditating, breathing in the frequencies of absolute trust and surrender to the perfection within our divinity.

Self–Healing Prayer Meditation: Example One (short form)

I love myself deeply.

I forgive myself for everything.

I forgive the world and all others for everything.

I trust and surrender to the Holy Spirit, the Light of my soul, to guide me, direct me, and heal me.

Thank you God for this blessing!

Self–Healing Prayer
Meditation: Example Two

In this version of the prayer, you are calling in the wisdom of God as it flows into you through your higher self as you say these lines:

I love myself completely, as I know you love me.

I forgive myself for everything, as you have shown me my innocence.

I forgive the world and all others, as you have shown me: we are all innocent.

I trust and surrender to the Divinity that dwells within me, to guide, direct, and free me of all self-imposed limitations and projections, that I may embody the Love that I am, in my every thought, word, and deed.

I give myself to love to show me how to live in perfect harmony with all in grace.

Thank you God for this wonderful blessing!

I release this prayer, and allow it to be so!

And so it is!

Praying Nonverbally to Heal the Body

Kahu Abraham explained that in ancient times, a kahuna would use the concept of family to communicate with the body, causing it to respond to their intentions. The tiny beings of your physical realm such as atoms and molecules are family; they will respond and unite as a family when you apply a specific quality of inclusion and direction, using Ha breathing. The breath becomes your prayer when it is combined with loving intentions. This is a way of praying that goes beyond words, for in this holy space of conscious awareness, you can telepathically communicate with the cells, the molecules, and atoms that make up all things. Kahu said:

> Unity wants to respond to unity, and love wants to
> respond to love." That same principle of attunement
> and family is also related to the physical body. The gods
> that ruled the forces of nature also ruled the cellular, the
> molecular, and atomic levels. It might be difficult for the
> modern world to understand that ancient people were
> concerned with molecular and atomic realms. When
> the missionaries came, they condemned the contact with
> all gods. However, the Hawaiians had both a scientific
> and spiritual connection to the elements, and believed
> the gods had vibrational influence over all life, from
> high above to far below. Therefore, kahuna were able to
> change structure by attuning themselves to these gods,
> having a communication with them to be able to do a

bone healing instantaneously or to be able to even bring a dead person back to life.

The body responds to the language of touch and motion. Simply touch your body with a gentle compassion, and begin to intuitively move your hands however they seem to want to move, and your vibrational prayers will be transmitted into the cells of the body. In this way, you're inviting the frequencies of love and unity into the molecules and atoms, raising their vibration to meet with you on a higher level. Molecules and atoms have memory and remember their proper alignment. Your loving touch with kind words (or thoughts) gently reminds them of their perfect alignment, allowing transformation to occur at a cellular level. Always bring affirmative confidence and loving passion to your thoughts and words for best results.

Ike Mana (Miracle Awareness): Who Am I as Awareness?

What if there was no separate self, no personality to compare with others? What if there was only a point of view—that is, "you" as the loving presence of awareness, witnessing everything as itself with no identification or meaning whatsoever, just your "point of you" being aware? Imagine resting, listening, feeling, touching, everything…as you, knowing you are not you but simply awareness itself. You are alive and at one with all that is—you simply are the spirit of awareness and as awareness, are given many gifts to share with your community. Be still and open your presence as you open your sacred heart. Allow the spirit of love to live through all your gifts; overflow and nourish everyone and all creation. Share your limitless goodness with and through all, influencing every aspect of your lifestream with loving kindness. Try this for one day, just moving through your day, not identifying with your personality or your chosen identities, but simply as awareness. Let your prayer be to meet everything and everyone without judgment, seeing them as they really are, through the eyes of an angel. Look at the ones you meet with compassion and a willingness to be present with them as awareness for just one day. You may begin to see everyone you meet in a different light, beyond their exterior and into their essence as living experiences of awareness.

Resolving Hurtful Projections in Relationships: Story by Wayne Kealohi Powell

While developing my healing practice, I was studying both A Course in Miracles (ACIM) and kahuna science—the way of aloha. I was in love with both systems; they validated ancient truths residing in my soul, allowing me to open a relationship with the Holy Spirit and my soul's authentic divinity. I was so excited about this that I wanted to share it with my mother, a devout Christian for whom the Holy Spirit was her best friend. One day I photocopied the first fifty-page introduction of ACIM on the topic "What is a Miracle?" and sent it to my mom. I thought she would love the Christian terms expressing how the Holy Spirit moves and blesses us. Just before I sealed the large envelope, I decided to throw in Serge King's *Little Pink Booklet of Aloha* to give the package a Hawaiian rainbow filled with wisdom and aloha light.

Two weeks later, I received in the mail a twelve-page, handwritten letter from my mother. She wrote that the principles of Huna were the work of the devil. She listed each principle, one at a time, and then listed at least a dozen bible verses that supported her projection after each principle, concluding at the end of all seven that I was going to hell for following the devil's work. I was deeply hurt by this projection because at that time, I was on a path that was leading me to become a minister of ancient sacred truths for the Church of the Holy Spirit–Spiritis Sancti. My mother never said a word about the fifty pages of ACIM that were written by the Holy Spirit—not one word! She only condemned with her Cuban passion in full force the *Little Pink Booklet of Aloha*. I was devastated, crushed, and bewildered.

A few years later, I fell very ill—so ill that I couldn't get out of bed. I couldn't eat and it was very difficult to walk to the bathroom without collapsing because my fever was so high. I felt like I was dying. As I lay there in bed, I reread the letter from my mother and cried. It hurt so much, not being validated by my own mother. We loved each other so much but were caught in a judgment projection loop. She saw me as misguided, not knowing the "real" God. I saw me as someone being totally guided by God, my first love. I was studying the "I am" presence teachings, kahuna science, and ACIM at that time. After a nasty bankruptcy and divorce with three children, these teachings were helping to distract my busy mind so my heart could begin healing. I found myself projecting onto her a judgment about how *she* saw me. I was projecting that she was blind and grossly misguided—not knowing the real God at all. These projections toward each other lasted for two years after sending her the ACIM package. So I prayed that day for resolution. In my vulnerability and weakness, I prayed for our relationship, for a miracle that love would somehow return to us. Here's what happened.

God (as guide or angel), gave me a clear vision with an explanation: "Follow the feeling of fear and condemnation you feel from your mother. Follow it and track it back to its source." I began to reflect how I had seen this pattern earlier in life; it happened with my first wife and I didn't know what to do then either. With my mom this time, I was determined to get it right. I followed her projection of condemnation and found that it led straight to her mind. This was no surprise to me because her words didn't feel loving. I said to God, "so what?" God said, "That's not where her projection originates from." He continued, "Follow it all the way to its origin." I hadn't noticed before that her mind was not where her projection began, because I was looking with *my* mind. My heart became curious so I followed her thoughts further and was led to her heart, of all places. This made absolutely no sense to me—how could judgment and condemnation come from her heart?

God showed me where the thought began in her heart: its origin was actually a purely loving thought, one of salvation for her son who she loved so much and wanted to see in Heaven one day after this world had released us both. She was trying to save me because it was how she was taught as a Christian to love me. When I saw how much my mother loved me from within her heart, my heart melted, and I had no more will to judge her for judging me. I saw her absolute innocence and was so in love with her, that I wrote her a letter on paper and sent it to her.

When she received the letter, she called me on the phone and left me a message. She was in tears while expressing her joy that she was going to see me, her son, in Heaven. Her new projection was that Jesus had "saved" me and now I would be going to Heaven. Now listen carefully: all I said in the letter was that I was overwhelmed by how much she loved me and that I felt so much love for her because of how deeply she cared for me in wanting me to go to Heaven when I die. I thanked her for being my mom and for all that she gave me as I was growing up. I showered her with gratitude from my heart overflowing.

We became so close; it was as if the condemnation had never happened at all. You see, what happened was the projection loop we were running with each other broke when I changed my focus and saw what was in her heart. Only then could I see clearly what was in my own. The belief systems we were running disappeared in the face of the brightest truth: "only love is real." —ACIM. This is an absolute truth; it doesn't change—it is true always and forever. Our hearts know this and thrive on its absolute strength to dissolve all suffering absolutely.

Projections are not real, plain and simple. The projection of condemnation from my mother was created in her mind by a limiting belief system. The love she holds for me was radically distorted by her beliefs as it rose from her heart and became filtered through her Christian ideals. All wars happen in this way. Men believe differently about something and choose to die attempting to validate its authenticity. There is always another way to pono! Shifting our perception of people regenerates *lokahi* (unity), within an upward spiral of gratitude for the good, the holy, and the beautiful to thrive in our lives.

Prayer to End Conflict and Release Projections

Say this prayer when caught in a conflict, a cycle of judgment with someone you care for very much. This is a call to your higher self to clear your projections and see the one before you as innocent. Perhaps they are coming from a place of distorted love, yet you know the love between you is the only thing that's real. And always remember that it only takes one to end a conflict between two or more, because everything you see, feel, and think is being generated by, and influenced within your own mind, *ike*. When you perceive something, you will tend to believe in what you perceived, so when you alter your perception, you will have an entirely different experience.

This prayer is used to stop yourself when you feel your judgments cloud your state of mind and need help from your higher self or the Holy Spirit to intervene and correct your thinking. We suggest hanging this on the refrigerator so when you forget to forgive, you'll have a handy reminder nearby. The kitchen area is the center of the house and where a lot of communication with family members happens. Conflict often ends up taking place here because conflict is a kind of food for relationships. We must learn to digest all the drama and trauma with our love. Without forgiveness, no real or lasting healing can actually take place. Remember to go vertical; say this prayer to your higher self. You are apologizing to your own divinity for judging another.

All Healing is Self-Healing

I have judged _____ (insert name of person or situation) as less than perfect.

I take full responsibility for this projection.

I am sorry. Please forgive me. (Now breathe vertically until you feel a change.)

I invite the Holy Spirit—the Light of my soul to correct my thinking,
shift my perception into seeing everyone's innocence,
and help me forgive myself for these hurtful projections.

I choose now to see the light of God in us all, now and always. (Now breathe vertically until you feel a shift in your energy aligning with Light.)

Thank you... I love you...

Affirmative Prayer
by Wayne Kealohi Powell

This short affirmative mantra is a song that was written as a declaration of purpose to remind us who we are, why we're here, and to be humble, forgiving, and authentic in all we do. You can sing your prayers in full voice when driving your car, walking in the woods, or taking a shower, imagining white light pouring into you. We invite you now to be the unique soul that you are, and let your light shine brightly, peacefully, and powerfully through all you do. Let your life become a thriving example of love in action. This is the greatest gift we can share with all those we love. This is a good mantra to say or sing in the shower every day!

Ke aloha o ke Akua (the grace of God)

I am the light of God that never fails

I am the love of God, in all prevails

I am the peace of God here to forgive

And in the grace of God forever live ...

CONCLUSION

You can always count on the authenticity of your own soul to attract the authenticity within the souls of others in all you do. If you move through life expressing your own authentic true self, you will always find support and encouragement from others who resonate with you along the way. The path of healing is unique for everyone, and you must do what is right for you. You cannot please everyone; when you follow your heart, you risk being judged for being different. When you don't play by the rules, you invite jealousy from the ones who do. Always do your best and then give it all up to source, allowing a higher authority to take over. Surrender. Thrive within all that you are truly, and share, share, share—it is why we came here, to thrive in love and extend our blessings to all beings.

Above all, remember that we are all in this together. None of us really knows what is going on, so a sense of humor can often be your greatest ally in all of life's circumstances. We all make mistakes, and we all get lost along the way. Let's allow ourselves to laugh, and as we see the humor in each situation, open to see more joy, light, innocence, and beauty. May the ancient rhythms of spirit in motion lift you, move through you, carry you, and guide your way home.

GLOSSARY

ahi: fire

ahonui: patience, tolerance

'a'i: neck

'aina: the spirit of the land

Aka: an energetic shadowy body that connects all things

akahai: careful offering, kindness, modesty, gentleness, tenderness, unpretentious, unassuming, unobtrusive

Akua: God or spirit (*akua nui*) great spirit

alaea: type of red clay gathered from specific locations on the Hawaiian Islands, very high in iron oxide *aloha:* this word embodies all the qualities of unconditional love, often used as an affectionate greeting between friends, family, or loved ones (aloha mana), miraculous power of unconditional love, (aloha nui), or great love

anuenue: rainbow

'ao: the light, the realm of spirit, similar to heaven, a place where many angelic spirits dwell

'awa: this is a sacred herb to the Hawaiian people, the root is drank ceremonially, also known as kava in other Pacific Islands

e kala mai: pardon me, excuse me, to ask for permission to enter, or to ask forgiveness

ha'aha'a: humble, modest

ha'i ha'i: the breaking-up massage for when the body is full of kinks and the nervous system needs adjustment

ha'i ha'i iwi: the Hawaiian practice of bone setting

halau: a collective of people who share in a particular body of knowledge or lineage passed down from one teacher, as in hula or lomilomi

Halawa Valley: a valley located on the island of Molokai

haole: a person not natively from Hawaii, especially a white person

haumana: a student who is dedicated to learning a specific body of knowledge *heiau:* a sacred ceremonial site or place reserved for specific people or the gods, often marked by rock walls and signs asking people not to enter or remove any rocks

helelena: face

hilina'i: trust

ho'iho'i: the replacement of organs that are out of position

hoku: star

honi: a kiss, in Hawaiian style, this is a form of greeting where noses are pressed side by side and breath is shared. The greeting where foreheads touch is a Maori form now used by many Hawaiians.

ho'omaika'i: to bring in goodness, to call in a blessing

ho'opono: to correct, or bring harmony

ho'oponopono: to make things right, a Hawaiian process for inner or outer conflict resolution, forgiveness, and bringing into right relationship

hula: type of dance originating from Hawaii

huli: to turn or flip over; to change

huna: hidden, or small; huna is the name given to the teachings of Hawaiian spirituality by Max Freedom Long, and later Serge Kahili King

'Iao Valley: A sacred valley on the island of Maui

'io: this is the word for the Hawaiian hawk, sometimes associated with our creator

'imua: to push forward, to charge ahead

iwi: bones

kahea: to sound a call

kahiko: the oldest form of hula, a story-telling dance

Kahi Loa: a style of shamanic bodywork taught by Serge Kahili King

kahu: a caretaker

kahuna: priest, magician, wizard, minister; an expert in a particular field or body of knowledge, such as fishing, navigating, or canoe building; one who gains mastery over the spiritual aspects of the work and spirituality as a way of life

kahuna la 'au kahea: a priest who heals with words

kai: the ocean water that is located near the shore

kala'e: to clear, as in removing stones from an irrigation ditch

kanaka maoli: native Hawaiians

Kane: a Hawaiian god associated with creation and the ocean; in Huna teachings, kane refers to the higher aspects of humanity's consciousness

kaona: the hidden meaning of a poem or a song

kapu: sacred; to keep out, or restricted

kaulike: to balance evenly; word used by Serge Kahili King for an energy balancing technique

keiki: child, offspring

kino: physical form, as in body

ku: to stand upright and erect; refers to the masculine principle a Hawaiian God associated with the primal aspects of man in huna teachings, (Ku) name given to the body mind, or the consciousness of the body

kuahu: altar

kuamo'o: spine

kuleana: a responsibility one has taken on and agreed to honor

kumu: this refers to the source of a body of knowledge, one's teacher or instructor

kupua: one possessing mana, special power, as a magician, shaman

kupuna: an esteemed elder

la'au: a leaf or a plant

la'au lapa'au: the use of plant medicines for healing

lani: the heavens

laulima: the practice of laying on of hands, often shared in a group for healing purposes

lokahi: unity

lomi: to knead or squeeze, as in massage

lomilomi: the practice of Hawaiian style massage

Lono: a Hawaiian god associated with peace and agriculture; in huna teachings, Lono is the name used when referring to one's conscious mind, the part of our mind that chooses which thoughts to focus on

Lua: Hawaiian martial arts

malama: to care for

mana: to possess personal power and have mastery over the life force energy

manahuna: "small power"; a name given to the native people who were smaller in stature inhabiting the islands when the Tahitians came to take over. The name later became *Menehune.*

manamana lima: hands and arms

mauli ola: the breath of life, the power of healing

Mo'oula Falls: a waterfall located in Halawa Valley on Molokai, named after the red dragon who watches over the falls

na'au: the intestines and the gut, the seat of feelings and emotions

na mea apau: everyone and everything

'ohana: family or extended family

oki: to cut

ola pau ole: eternal life

'olelo: story or language

oli: chant

'olu'olu: pleasing, pleasant

'opu: stomach

pa'a: solid, to hold firm, can also be used to speak of holding one's focus in the present moment *papakole:* hips

pau: finished

pilikia: trouble of any kind

po: the dark, the realm of the unmanifest, from where life comes forth

pohaku: stone

po'o: head

po'ohiwi: shoulders

pule: prayer

pule o'o: powerful prayers

pu'uwai: the heart center

'uhane: in huna teachings it is the soul of the mind/conscious awareness, associated with your spirit/soul, which can travel during dreamtime, or become a ghost

'unihipili: in huna teachings it is the soul/consciousness of the body, associated with the spirit leaving the body at the time of death

'uniki: spiritual ordination, validating your entry into the healing modality

Wai: fresh water, liquid or blood

wawae: feet and legs

SPIRITUAL TERMS

adamantine particles: particles which manifest and delineate infinity, activating its potential and making possible all manifest form

bone washing: cleaning and clearing the skin of the bones, removing density or crystallized energies, from the joints out the extremities

Christ: the perfection within each of us that has been anointed by the spirit of love. Embodying a highly quantified, potent ray of divinity, known as the aloha spirit, from a New Age perspective, Christ is seen as living inside of us; a spirit that has awakened within us, as us and for us, the qualities of divine love.

creating space: creating space between the bones and joints of the body through the use of lifting, wiggling, shaking, pulling, and pounding in connection with breathing fully and deeply—releasing during a full exhale

elemental beings: the spirits of the elements that dwell in nature

elements: the basic building blocks of life—earth, air, fire, and water

enlightenment: a state of expansion and heightened awareness of oneness with all life, with God, and mastery over states of consciousness

entity: an energetic form or a fragmented aspect of a soul that can become attached to someone's energy field

giver: refers to the person giving a healing treatment

God: the indescribable, omnipotent, omnipresent spirit of love, harmony, beauty, and perfection that runs through all life, the creative aspect of our existence

god/goddess: icons and archetypes used by ancient people to call upon, connect, and bring awareness to various aspects of the divine

Ha breath medicine: uses the breath to transmute and clear stuck energy, releasing emotional blockages, and transforming expired contracts with self and others

healer: a person who can assist another to create a shift of energy that can bring about positive change *healing:* a shift of energy that can be integrated into the physical, mental, and spiritual aspects of oneself, bringing positive change on all levels; returning to wholeness

Heartworks: the name given to Sherman Dudoit by his teacher to use for the lineage of traditional lomi that he carried

I Am: used to describe that part of us that is a witness, our higher self; the part of us that remains united with God, the Divine, and all life. This term became well known when the "I Am" discourses were written in the 1930s by Geoffrey King.

kingdoms of nature: main types of life that exist on Earth—Plant, Animal, Human

lost soul: a fragmentation of soul in which parts of a soul become trapped in other times or dimensions, a ghost that is trapped on the earthly plane

Mu: an ancient continent that once existed (now lies below the water) in the Pacific Ocean

receiver: refers to the person receiving a healing treatment

shaman: one who works with the forces of nature and the spirit world to bring change or transformation to themselves, their environment, and to others

Shamanic Bodywork: the traveling mystery school created and founded by Kumu Wayne Powell

Soul: the integration of one's being, in conscious energetic form, unifying body, mind, and spirit

soul retrieval: type of healing experience in which one reconnects to aspects of their soul that have become energetically damaged because of trauma, and integrates them within their energetic field of awareness. Issues from past lives can be resolved, bringing resolution to the issues in this lifetime

Spirit: our awareness; the divine spark within each of us, which can enter or leave the body and lives on beyond the body after physical death

violet flame: from the "I Am" Discourses, and refers to a cleansing energetic "flame" that can be called upon and used for clearing, energetic purification, and healing

ACKNOWLEDGMENTS

We give thanks to our teachers who shared aloha so freely on our path of discovery, practice, and teaching of Hawaiian Healing and include: Serge Kahili King, for his knowledge of the Hawaiian language, philosophy, and history and inspiring us to share kahuna science with the world; Harry Uhane Jim, who brought us his divine flavor of "easy" aloha, empowered with kahuna wisdom and sublime, effective Hawaiian healing techniques; Sherman Raman Das Dudoit brought the essence of advaita, meditation, stillness, sweetness, and gentle, egoless presence into our work with Heartworks Lomi; Abraham Kawai'i inspired us to go beyond our limitations fearlessly in every way in order to lift up others with our teachings, open our wings and fly; Anakala Pilipo Solatorio for connecting us to the roots of the 'aina and people of Molokai and sharing the priceless gift of aloha, 'ohana, and pono in Halawa Valley; Susan Pa'iniu Floyd introduced Temple Style Lomi, sparking us to grow into Hawaiian Shamanic Bodywork; Aunty Mahealani O Henry, the Aloha Aunty, for sharing aloha and mana'o about Hawaiian traditions and ancestral wisdom and how they relate to our lives today; Kim and Jim Hartley, wise and devoted lomi teachers who with so much care and love taught the Aunty Margaret traditional Big Island massage routine; Mahara Brenna for sharing her remarkable way of healing, lifting cherished wounds through "breath work" and her profound connection to the angelic realm; Lawrence Kamani Aki introduced us to Anakala Pilipo and his 'ohana in Halawa Valley on Molokai, both with such dedication to preserving the traditions and history of Molokai, and sharing the traditional form of Ho'oponopono and Kava ceremony; Lono and his Halau for sharing Hawaiian history, stories, music, and hula of Molokai; Dhyana Ahiwai Bartkow for teaching the sacred dance of hula.

We give thanks to our team who helped shape this book into form with their profound gifts and generous hearts: Kate Osborne, our fearless and awesome editor in chief, who was our constant companion and confident guide through this amazing journey; Cynthia Davis, who assisted Wayne in becoming a writer in the true sense of the word, opening the way for the beginning of this long, incredible process to unfold; Gary Dillon, for his unique point of view on Wayne's writing, helping us to expand our perspective on our ideas in many wonderful ways; Karen La Verne, who proofread every word and loved and supported us, giving of herself, opening her heart and her home when we needed it most to complete this journey.

BIBLIOGRAPHY

Chai, R. Makana Risser. *Na Mo'olelo Lomilomi*. Honolulu, HI: Bishop Museum, 2005.

Cowan, Eliot. *Plant Spirit Medicine*. Columbus, NC: Swan Raven & Co, 1995.

Green, Glenda. *Love Without End: Jesus Speaks*. Sedona, AZ: Spiritis Publishing, 1998.

Hrehorczak-Stephens, Tamara. *Abraham Kawai'i: A Brief History of the Man, the Kahuna, and Kahuna Bodywork*. Charleston, SC: CreateSpace Publishing, 2012.

Jim, Harry Uhane. *Wise Secrets of Aloha*. San Francisco, CA: Red Wheel Weiser, 2007.

Joseph, Jeshua ben. *The Way of Mastery: The Way of the Heart, The Way of Transformation, The Way of Knowing*. Sacramento, CA: The Shanti Christo Foundation, 2004.

King, Serge Kahili. *Huna: Ancient Hawaiian Secrets for Modern Living.* Neptune City, NJ: Beyond Words, 2008.

Lee, Pali Jai. *Tales from the Night Rainbow.* Honolulu, HI: Night Rainbow Publishing Co, 1990.

Osho. *Osho Zen Tarot.* New York: Osho International Foundation, 1994.

Pukui, Mary Kawena. *Hawaiian Dictionary.* Honolulu, HI: University of Hawaii Press, 1986.

Wesselman, Hank. *Bowl of Light.* Louisville, CO: Sounds True Publishing, 2011.

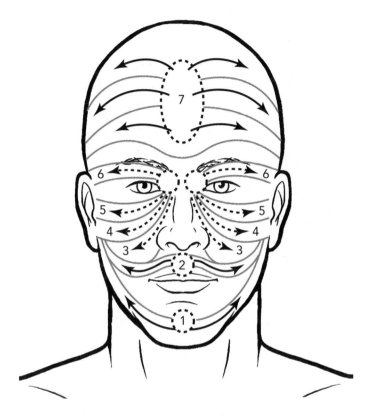

Bonewashing the face.

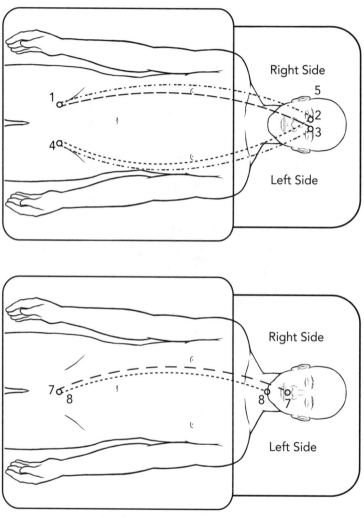

Balancing the neurological circuits.

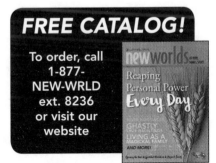

KRISTIN MADDEN

THE BOOK OF
SHAMANIC
HEALING

INCLUDES TECHNIQUES FOR BREATHING,
DREAM WORK, DRUMMING, AND SOUL RETRIEVAL

The Book of Shamanic Healing
Kristin Madden

Here is everything a shaman healer needs in his or her tool-kit. Shamanism is an all-encompassing lifestyle of deep self-knowledge and powerful healing. In this groundbreaking book, a modern shaman gives the practitioner concrete advice and ideas on several aspects of shamanic healing. You will learn to prepare yourself for healing work, communicate with spirit guides, free your voice and seek your power song, safely explore your shadow side, partner with your drum to create healing, and heal yourself and others. The author also covers practical ethical matters such as taking payment and working with friends.

978-0-7387-0271-1, 264 pp., 6 x 9   **$16.99**

To order, call 1-877-NEW-WRLD
Prices subject to change without notice
Order at Llewellyn.com 24 hours a day, 7 days a week!

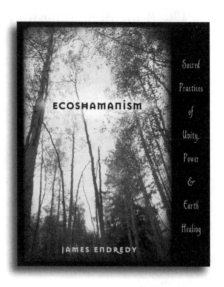

ECOSHAMANISM

Sacred
Practices
of
Unity,
Power
&
Earth
Healing

JAMES ENDREDY

Ecoshamanism
Sacred Practices of Unity, Power & Earth Healing
James Endredy

James Endredy, who has studied with tribal shamans all over the world, offers a rigorous and authentic new philosophy of shamanic practice called ecoshamanism. Rejecting the consumer/industrial worldview and the spiritual deadness that accompanies it, ecoshamanism leads to a fundamental shift in consciousness-first, by becoming aware of the sacred natural world and our role within it, and next, by forging a spiritual alliance with the sentient forces that sustain our planet. Using the powerful ceremonies, sacred rituals, and everyday practices in this guidebook, you can transform your life as you save the world.

978-0-7387-0742-6, 360 pp., 7½ x 9⅛   **$26.95**

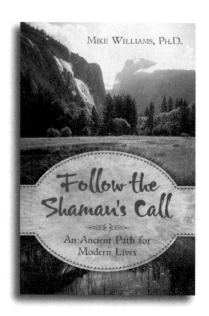

MIKE WILLIAMS, PH.D.

Follow the
Shaman's Call

An Ancient Path for
Modern Lives

Follow the Shaman's Call
An Ancient Path for Modern Lives
MIKE WILLIAMS

This evocative and experiential guide reveals how you can immediately begin to transform your life by following the path of the shaman. Author Mike Williams, Ph.D., presents hands-on exercises and engaging true stories from decades of shamanic practice and academic study into ancient European traditions.

Once you understand the powerful forces of the unseen world, you'll learn how to apply the tenets of shamanism to your own life in a variety of practical ways: predicting the future and understanding the past, using dreamwork to find answers to problems, and clearing your house of negativity. You'll discover how to find your power animal and meet your spirit guides, journey to the otherworlds for healing and self-empowerment, and live in harmony with the world.

978-0-7387-1984-9, 264 pp., 6 x 9   **$17.99**

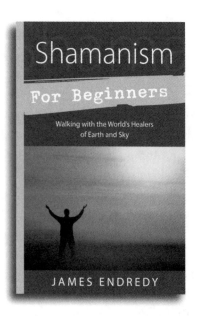

Shamanism

For Beginners

Walking with the World's Healers
of Earth and Sky

JAMES ENDREDY

Shamanism for Beginners
Walking with the World's Healers of Earth and Sky
JAMES ENDREDY

Healers and visionaries, food-finders and rainmakers—as intermediaries between the physical and spirit worlds, shamans have served a vital role in indigenous cultures for more than 40,000 years. The timeless wisdom of the shaman also holds relevance for the challenges we face today.

James Endredy explores shamanic paths from around the globe and discusses the tools, rituals, and beliefs that are common to most traditions. You'll discover how shamans are chosen and initiated, and how they establish a relationship with power animals, ancestors, and other inhabitants of the spirit realm. Along with many stories from his own experiences, Endredy shares insights from other scholars in the field, including Mircea Eliade, Michael Harner, and Holger Kalweit, and from indigenous shamans throughout history.

Shamanism for Beginners concludes with a thoughtful, empowering look at how shamanic practices can help restore balance and peace to our lives and the earth.

978-0-7387-1562-9, 288 pp., 5³⁄₁₆ x 8   **$14.95**

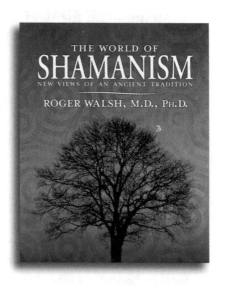

THE WORLD OF

SHAMANISM

NEW VIEWS OF AN ANCIENT TRADITION

ROGER WALSH, M.D., Ph.D.

The World of Shamanism
New Views of an Ancient Tradition
Roger Walsh

Many of the books on shamanism are either decades old, simply repeat what is in those books, or are of questionable accuracy. Now, scholar, researcher, and professor Roger Walsh—whose writings and research have received over two dozen national and international awards and honors—presents new views and studies on the oldest spiritual traditions in *The World of Shamanism.*

This book is simply the most complete volume that provides an overview of shamanism, its practices, techniques, beliefs, and effects. But it is far more than that. It also examines all of the techniques, using modern research to determine two things: Do they really work? And if so, why do they work?

978-0-7387-0575-0, 336 pp., 7½ x 9⅛   **$21.99**

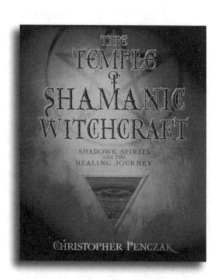

THE
TEMPLE
OF
SHAMANIC
WITCHCRAFT

SHADOWS, SPIRITS
AND THE
HEALING JOURNEY

CHRISTOPHER PENCZAK

The Temple of Shamanic Witchcraft
Shadows, Spirits, and the Healing Journey
CHRISTOPHER PENCZAK

Is shamanism all that different from modern witchcraft? According to Christopher Penczak, Wicca's roots go back 20,000 years to the Stone Age shamanic traditions of tribal cultures worldwide. A fascinating exploration of the Craft's shamanic origins, *The Temple of Shamanic Witchcraft* offers year-and-a-day training in shamanic witchcraft.

Penczak's third volume of witchcraft teachings corresponds to the water element—guiding the reader into this realm of emotion, reflection, and healing. The twelve formal lessons cover shamanic cosmologies, journeying, dreamwork, animal/plant/stone medicine, totems, soul retrieval, and psychic surgery. Each lesson includes exercises (using modern techniques and materials), assignments, and helpful tips. The training ends with a ritual for self-initiation into the art of the shamanic witch—culminating in an act of healing, rebirth, and transformation.

978-0-7387-0767-9, 480 pp., 7½ x 9⅛　　　　**$22.99**
